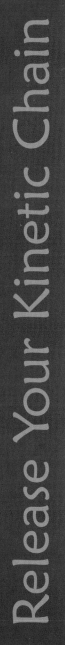

Release Your Kinetic Chain

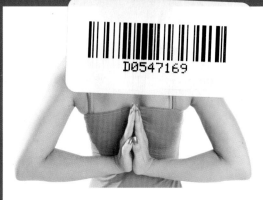

D0547169

Exercises for the Shoulder to Hand

Activating Your Arm's Kinetic Chain!

Dr. Brian James Abelson, DC, ART
Kamali T. Abelson, B.Sc.

Kinetic Health
Calgary, Alberta, Canada

Kinetic chain exercises for the
Release Your Body
series of books

Canadian Cataloguing in Publication Data
Abelson, Brian and Abelson, Kamali
Exercises for the Shoulder to Hand© **Volume 2 of Release Your Kinetic Chain**
Includes index and glossary.

Copyright Registration	1071569
ISBN-13 - Hardcopy	978-0-9733848-6-4
ISBN-13 - E-Copy	978-0-9733848-7-1

First Printing: 2010, Rowan Tree Books Ltd.
Printed in USA 10 9 8 7 6 5 4 3 2 1

Notice: Although the authors, editors, and publishers have made every effort to ensure the accuracy and completeness of information contained in this book, it is difficult to ensure that all of the information is accurate, and the possibility of error can never be completely eliminated. The authors, editors, and publishers disclaim any liability or responsibility for injury or damage to persons or property, that is incurred as a consequence, directly or indirectly, of the use and application of any of the contents of this book, as well as for any unintentional slights to any person or entity.

Credits
Production and Editing: Kamali Abelson, Hannah MacLeod
Technical Editors: Dr. Brian J. Abelson, Dr. Tarveen Ahluhwalia
Illustrations: Lavanya Balasubramanian, 123RF Limited, Rowan Tree Books Ltd.
Cover artwork by: Studio Sun

Certain images and/or photos in this book are the copyrighted property of 123RF Limited, its Contributors or Licensed Partners and are being used with permission under license. These images and/or photos may not be copied or downloaded without permission from 123RF Limited.

The Publishers have made every effort to trace the copyright holders for borrowed materials. If they have inadvertently overlooked any, they will be pleased to make the necessary arrangements at the first opportunity.

Kinetic Health books are available at a special discount for bulk purchase by practitioners, corporations, institutions, and other organizations. For details, see our website or contact the Special Sales Manager at Kinetic Health.

Kinetic Health® **Web Sites**:
> www.releaseyourbody.com
> www.drabelson.com
> www.activerelease.ca

Canada: **Kinetic Health**®
        Edgemont Chiropractic - Soft-tissue Management Systems
        34 Edgedale Drive N.W.
        Calgary, AB, Canada, T3A 2R4
        403-241-3772 (bus)
        403-241-3846 (fax)

Health Disclaimer

This book provides wellness management in an informational and educational manner only, with information that is general in nature and that is not specific to you, the reader. The contents of this book are intended to assist you and other readers in your personal wellness efforts.

Nothing in this book should be construed as personal advice or diagnosis, and must *not* be used in this manner. The information provided about conditions is general in nature. This information does not cover all possible uses, actions, precautions, side-effects, or interactions of medicines, or medical procedures. The information in this book should not be considered as complete and does *not* cover all diseases, ailments, physical conditions, or their treatment.

You should consult with your physician before beginning any exercise, weight loss, or health care program. This book should *not* be used in place of a call or visit to a competent health-care professional. You should consult a health care professional before adopting any of the suggestions in this book or before drawing inferences from it. Any decision regarding treatment and medication for your condition should be made with the advice and consultation of a qualified health care professional. If you have, or suspect you have, a health-care problem, then you should immediately contact a qualified health care professional for treatment.

Exercise Disclaimer

For Details: See "Exercise Disclaimer...Please read!" on page xi.

No Warranties

The authors, publishers, and/or their respective directors, shareholders, officers, employees, agents, trainers, contractors, representatives, successors do not guarantee or warrant the quality, accuracy, completeness, timeliness, appropriateness or suitability of the information in this book, or of any product or services referenced by this book. The information in this book is provided on an "as is" basis and the authors and publishers make no representations or warranties of any kind with respect to this information. This book may contain inaccuracies, typographical errors, or other errors.

Liability Disclaimer

The publishers, authors, and any other parties involved in the creation, production, provision of information, or delivery of this book specifically disclaim any responsibility, and shall not be liable for any damages, claims, injuries, losses, liabilities, costs or obligations including any direct, indirect, special, incidental, or consequential damages (collectively known as "Damages") whatsoever and howsoever caused, arising out of, or in connection with, the use or misuse of the book and the information contained within it, whether such Damages arise in contract, tort, negligence, equity, statute law, or by way of any other legal theory. x

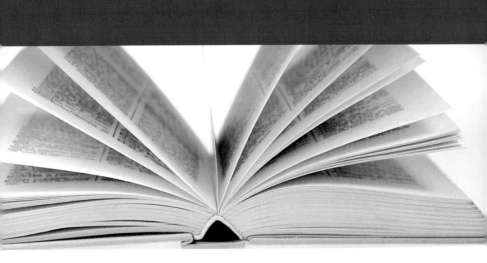

Table of Contents

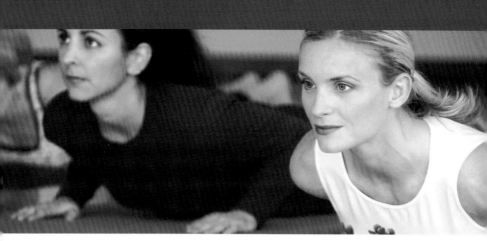

Exercise Disclaimer...Please read!

Exercise is not without its risks, and this or any other exercise program may result in injury. Risks include but are not limited to: aggravation of a pre-existing condition, risk of injury, or adverse effects of over-exertion such as muscle strain, abnormal blood pressure, fainting, disorders of heartbeat, and in very rare instances, of heart attack.

To reduce the risk of injury in your case, consult your doctor before beginning this exercise program. The instruction and advice presented here are in no way intended as a substitute for medical consultation. The authors and publisher disclaim any liability from and in connection with this program.

The exercises in this book are provided for educational purposes only, and are not to be interpreted as a recommendation for a specific treatment plan, product, or course of action, or as a substitute for professional supervision or advice. To reduce the risk of injury in your case, consult your doctor before beginning this or any exercise program.

The authors, publishers, and technical experts use reasonable effort to include accurate and up-to-date information in its information sources; however, all information appearing is general in nature. Kinetic Health, the authors, publishers, and practitioners do not assume liability or give any warranty of any kind for the information and data contained or omitted from this document or for any action or inaction made in reliance thereon. Information presented in this book and associated web sites may be changed at any time. Specific advice should be obtained in respect of specific situations.

Any programs involving weights, intense workouts and apparatus may put strong physical demands on any child who is still growing – supervision is obligatory in such cases. If you have or have had asthma, growth condition, heart condition, or have experienced chest pains or dizziness in the last month we strongly advise you NOT to try any of our workouts. This book is NOT a medical facility and no information contained in our book should be used to prevent, treat or diagnose medical conditions of any kind. As with any exercise program, if at any point during your workout you begin to feel faint, dizzy, or have physical discomfort, you should stop immediately and consult a physician.

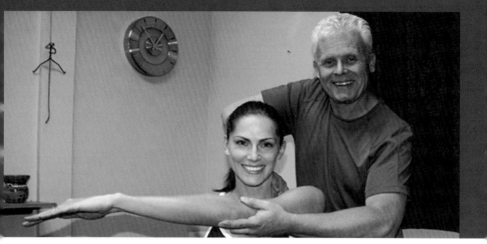

Foreword by Dr. Brian Abelson

All too often, we find our patients and athletes jumping into the advanced, intensive stages of exercise before establishing needed ground work. This rushed approach leads to more injuries and an accompanying lack of performance.

The **Release Your Kinetic Chain** series of exercise books takes a **functional** approach to exercise. With this approach, we give you step-by-step recommendations to help you move through the **rehabilitation phase** of an exercise program to prepare you for the **performance phase**.

This book (and its sister books) have two basic objectives:

- The first objective is to help you rehabilitate your body after an injury (or long period of inactivity) and prepare it for more intensive exercise programs.

- The second objective is to help you prepare your body so that it is ready for sport or athletic performance training.

Rehabilitating an Injury...do this first!

There are some basic concepts that you need to understand in order to be successful with our program. First of all, when you are rehabilitating an injury, we will always have you work in a completely **pain-free zone**. That's right...at this phase, the concept of *no pain, no gain* is completely wrong! Our primary objective with rehabilitation is to increase muscular endurance and neurological motor control. With rehabilitation routines, we always work within a pain-free zone...essentially a zone of safety where you can bring your injured areas back to normal activity.

Our family of exercise books focuses on exercise routines that help you to rehabilitate your body from previous injuries, and bring it up to speed for the next phase of performance training. Your injury could be as minor as an ankle sprain, or more substantial such as recovery from a surgery! In all cases, it is critical that you take your body through the rehabilitative exercise phase before jumping into the performance phase!

You will find that the Beginner and Intermediate routines expect you to work within this pain-free rehabilitative zone. The Advanced routines will help to transition you into the Performance or Athletic arenas.

Increasing Your Performance...wait to do this!

Only **after** you have established good muscle endurance and motor control (neurological control) should you focus upon increasing your strength or speed.

Increasing strength should only come after good neuromuscular endurance has been established. If you try to increase strength too quickly, you will discover that you have found the best formula for **developing ongoing injuries**.

In this book, we provide proven exercise routines that gradually build your strength and endurance to the point where you will be ready to begin performance training.

Why you need these books

The training programs in these books are very different from the body-building type of programs you will find in most gyms. The purpose of most body-building programs is to increase the *size* of individual body parts – that is, to develop a state of muscle hypertrophy. Body-building often trains the body, not as a set of linked kinetic chains, but as a series of unconnected segments.

This type of training can be a major mistake when you are trying to rehabilitate an injury or when you are trying to improve your sports performance. Often these body-building programs create muscle imbalances, cause even more injuries in unprepared tissues, and result in an overall decrease in performance. This is a huge price to pay, even if your initial goal was to simply increase muscle size by isolating and growing specific muscle groups.

Instead, the exercise programs in the *Release Your Kinetic Chain* book series use step-by-step procedures which take into consideration kinetic chain relationships, tissue interactions, core imbalances, elastic power, and aerobic training. We strive to give you a balanced means of achieving a good strong body that is injury-free.

■ Our exercise routines always take into consideration a key fundamental aspect of good rehabilitation – **Kinetic Chain Relationships.** Since injury or weakness in one area of your body always affects the function of numerous other related areas, we ensure that our routines take into account direct muscular connections, muscle antagonists, fascial connections, as well as the fact that tissue restrictions affect the primary mechanisms of energy storage and release. See *"Shoulder to Hand – a Kinetic Chain" on page 31.*

■ Our exercise routines always consider how the core of your body acts as the power generator for your entire body. This is true even for movements of your neck, shoulders, arms, hands, legs or feet. No matter what the action, you need a strong stable core to be able to transfer energy to your extremities. *See "Involving Your Core" on page 22.*

■ Our exercise routines also address the development of your elastic power or the ability of your muscles, ligaments, tendons, and fascia to store and release energy. The ability of your soft tissues to store and release energy is dependent upon the quality of your soft tissues. Low-quality tissues are full of adhesions, scar tissues, and knots. These tissues do not store or release energy efficiently. High-quality tissues can move easily through their full range of motion, are not restricted or adhesed, are capable of long periods of endurance, and are not easily injured. One of the primary goals of our exercise routines is to provide you with a means for improving your overall tissue quality. See *"Principle 2: Good Tissue Quality = Good Performance" on page 12.*

- Aerobic warm-ups are an integral component of all of our programs. It doesn't matter if we are dealing with a jaw, neck, shoulder, back, or leg injury; aerobic training is essential. By developing your aerobic system you increase your circulatory function and your ability to produce energy on demand. Aerobic exercise does this by increasing the density of capillaries in your muscles, and the density of mitochondria (your personal energy factories) in your cells. See *"Improving Cellular Function with Aerobic Exercises" on page 17.*

- And finally, one of our primary goals is to give you effective strategies for increasing strength without further injuring yourself. The exercise routines we provide in these books are similar to ones that we provide to our patients. These routines have been successfully tested and improved over time, and will help you to strengthen your body in a gentle and progressive manner.

I hope you stick to the routines, enjoy this book, and benefit from your improved health. I am sure you will achieve great results.

All the best in health!

Dr. Brian Abelson

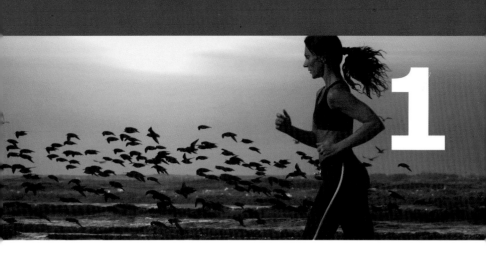

Rehabilitating an Injury

When you are looking for resolution from injuries, restrictions, or reduced function, you should always ensure that your solution takes into account the kinetic chain for that structure.

People often assume that their injury occurred at the time that they first noticed symptoms (pain, discomfort, or inability to perform an action), but this is often not the case. Other than when an injury is caused by acute trauma, the actual cause of many injuries is often unknown. This is due to the slow insidious nature of many soft-tissue injuries.

With many injuries, symptoms (pain and discomfort) are often the very last thing to surface. In actuality, the conditions that led to the injury may have existed for a long time before the symptoms manifested. In some cases, our patients have undergone years of micro-trauma before the first noticeable symptom appeared.

For example, if you injure a muscle in your arm, your body immediately compensates by using surrounding structures to *support*, and sometimes to *perform*, the activity that is normally carried out by this muscle. This compensation may initially only affect the surrounding muscles, ligaments, tendons, and connective tissues.

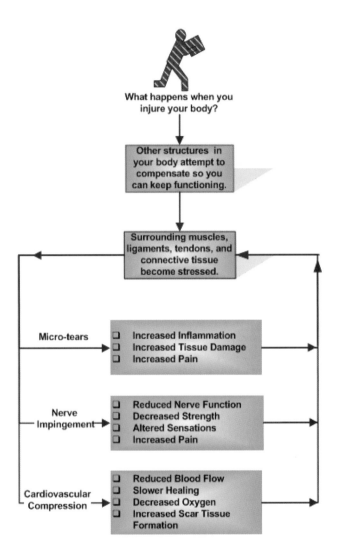

What happens when you
injure your body?

Other structures in
your body attempt to
compensate so you
can keep functioning.

Surrounding muscles,
ligaments, tendons, and
connective tissue
become stressed.

Micro-tears

- ❏ Increased Inflammation
- ❏ Increased Tissue Damage
- ❏ Increased Pain

Nerve
Impingement

- ❏ Reduced Nerve Function
- ❏ Decreased Strength
- ❏ Altered Sensations
- ❏ Increased Pain

Cardiovascular
Compression

- ❏ Reduced Blood Flow
- ❏ Slower Healing
- ❏ Decreased Oxygen
- ❏ Increased Scar Tissue
  Formation

Problems arise when the initial injury does not resolve, causing the
supporting structures to also become stressed or injured. This
creates a cycle of ongoing compensations which in turn leads to
reduced neurological function (due to impingement upon
neurological structures) and increased inflammation (due to
increased biomechanical tension, micro-tears, and inflammation).

The Cumulative Injury Cycle

One of the best explanations of this ongoing injury process was first postulated by Dr. Michael Leahy, the developer of Active Release Techniques® (ART), in his *Cumulative Injury Cycle*[1]. The Cumulative Injury Cycle describes the major factors that lead to the initial injury, and explains how these injuries are perpetuated.

Whether the injury is the result of an acute trauma, repetitive motions (RSI injuries), or internal tissue pressure, the result is often the same.

Each of these factors leads to a proliferation of fibrous tissue (scar tissue). Once this fibrous tissue forms, muscles become weaker, friction increases, inflammation increases, oxygen transport and distribution diminishes, and a cycle of dysfunction is created.

What Can You Do About This?

Fortunately, there is a lot you can do to break this cycle of injury. The initial phase of an injury is known as the ***Inflammatory Phase***. With acute injuries, R.I.C.E should be used within the first 48 to 72 hours.

- **R** = **Rest** to prevent further damage. But not too long a rest as immobilization can result in scar formation. See *Benefits of Rest - page 217* for more information.

- **I** - **Ice** to reduce swelling, inflammation, and pain. See *Cold Therapy - page 212* for more information.

- **C** = **Compression** to provide support, reduce swelling, and reduce bleeding.

- **E** = **Elevate** the injured area above the heart-level to reduce swelling and bleeding.

Without exercise, the probability of the collagen being laid down in a random manner and forming scar tissue is very high. Scar tissue is limited in its function, reduces movement, decreases circulation, and reduces sensation. The greater the amount of scar tissue, the

---

1. Cumulative Injury Cycle, Dr. P. Michael Leahy, Active Release Techniques Soft Tissue Management Systems for the Upper Extremity, 2nd Edition, 2008

greater the reduction in function of your muscles and other soft-tissues.

Injury Recovery

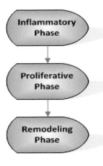

The second phase of injury recovery is known as *Proliferative Phase* and is characterized by the laying down of new collagen. This phase can start within two days of the injury and can last up to six weeks.

It is extremely important to be exercising during the Proliferative Phase as this will ensure that new collagen is laid down in the same fibre orientation as your muscle tissue, and that the new collagen does not inhibit relative motion between tissue layers.

The third and final stage of injury recovery is known as the *Remodeling Phase* and can last from three weeks to twelve months. During this phase the new collagen fibres remodel in proportion to the stress placed upon them. It is critical that you continue to exercise during this phase or your collagen fibres will never remodel fully.

So when injury strikes, do not pick and choose your exercises. We have designed our exercise routines to take you through these phases while addressing the needs of your entire kinetic chain. These programs will help you strengthen and heal – not just the initial area of pain, but also all the surrounding supportive soft-tissues in that structure's kinetic chain.

Do these exercises when you find your hands and arms becoming stiff and restricted, to restore the mobility and function of your muscles and joints. Do the **stretches** whenever you are spending long hours in front of a computer keyboard! And do the **strengthening** exercises to resolve or prevent injuries, and improve your performance in all your activities.

During all injury recovery phases, soft-tissue manipulation such as Active Release Techniques or Massage Therapy can be very effective in reducing muscle spasms, reducing swelling, decreasing nerve compression, and reducing pain.

Rehabilitation vs. Athletic Training

A Kinetic Chain Perspective

Exercise protocols and training methods should be quite different when you are rehabilitating an injury to bring your body up to a functional level of activity vs. when you are striving to improve athletic performance on an already well-trained, uninjured body. After all, the goals and capabilities of the trainee are quite different within the two levels of training.

Unfortunately, most standard exercise programs do not differentiate between the two goals, and tend to apply the same exercise routines in both situations. Moving too fast, with an unprepared body, into athletic or performance training is a sure recipe for injury and disaster.

The objective of our *Release Your Kinetic Chain* series of exercise books is to provide exercises that help you resolve injuries in specific areas of your body, and to prepare your body for the more difficult performance-based workouts. These books provide a step-by-step, methodical process, that requires patience and time, on your part.

Let's take a few minutes to understand the difference between these two types of programs – *Rehabilitative* and *Athletic* Training.

About Rehabilitative Exercise Routines

Rehabilitation programs focus upon returning your body to a state of full function without further injuring yourself in the process. Our primary objective with our rehabilitation programs is to resolve your injury, increase neurological and motor control, build strength, and increase flexibility while restoring function.

Only after you have rehabilitated completely from an injury, and have restored good muscle endurance and motor control (neurological control) should you consider applying athletic performance strategies to your training.

Rehabilitation training is not just for resolving existing injuries, it is also a critical preliminary step for preparing your body to accept and benefit from advanced conditioning and performance training. If you have not been physically active for a period of time, it is essential that you start with the *Beginner* sections of this book. As you work your way through the exercise levels, you will be tuning and preparing your body for more advanced performance-based exercises.

Rehabilitaton requires patience and time! Remember, your body needs time to heal from your injuries. Many people, in their enthusiasm to reach their goal, make their injuries worse by not giving their body sufficient time to heal. So take the time to properly prepare your body for athletic level training.

What we provide in these books are guidelines for gently tuning your body without causing undue stress, injury, or pain! But it is your responsibility to *listen to your body, understand its signals,* and adjust your routines accordingly.

The following rules are a few fundamental principles that you should keep in mind as you work through your rehabilitative routines:

- *Principle 1: No Pain...All Gain! - page 6.*
- *Principle 2: Develop your Power - page 7.*
- *Principle 3: Build your Aerobic Base - page 9.*

Principle I: No Pain...All Gain!

Conventional rehabilitation strategies commonly do not succeed because they do not address the underlying neuromuscular problems. They are often designed to make you work through your pain (as in work-hardening programs). This only causes you to create or reinforce the abnormal motor responses which in turn continues to keep you in pain.

In addition, if you work through pain caused by tissue damage you run the risk of *central sensitization*. This is a nervous system process which causes you to become more sensitive to pain. The only way to break this pattern is to perform your exercises in a pain-free zone. We commonly have patients come to our clinic who have exercised through their pain for years! They are always amazed at how, by exercising within a pain-free zone, we were able to help them break their pain-cycle in just a few short weeks.

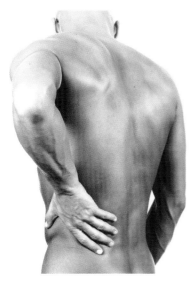

Rehabilitation (unlike athletic training) requires that you perform your exercises within a *completely pain-free* zone; essentially, a *zone of safety.*

Exercising in a manner that causes pain develops abnormal neuromuscular patterns that may lead to further injury.

If you truly want to rehabilitate your injuries you must work within a **pain-free** zone. This is quite different from training to improve your performance in which you may have to endure some degree of muscle pain (not injury pain) to improve strength and endurance.

Bottom line: *Never work through injury pain.* If you have an injury, and the exercise hurts during certain motions, or if you feel pain when resting, then restrict the range of motion of the exercise to lie within your pain-free range. In addition, avoid the exercises that currently cause you pain, until your body is ready for them.

What works will vary from person to person so *listen to your body* and adjust our routines accordingly.

Principle 2: Develop your Power

Power (within your body) is about the production and transfer of force through your entire body. Power is also a function of how well you can recruit your nervous system to control muscular action.

The more efficient your nervous system, the more power you will have. The more power you have, the easier it is to perform your activities and exercises without injury.

Power is not the same as strength; power is about maximum efficiency without effort. (Strength requires a lot of effort and energy.) The more power you have, the less energy you will need to expend to perform a task, which equates to having more energy available to heal and grow your body.

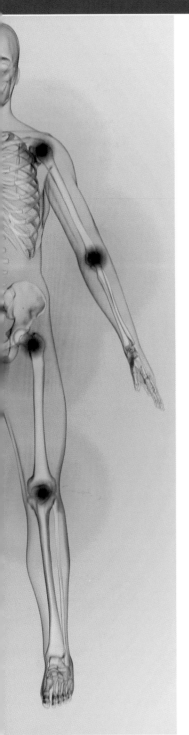

Power generation is also directly related to the **quality** of your soft tissues (muscles, ligaments, tendons, etc.). The quality of your soft tissues determines how well you can store and release energy.

Think of your soft tissues as being like cords of elastic rubber (or perhaps a telephone cord) that can stretch (storing energy) and contract (releasing energy). In a healthy state, your muscles contract and release instantaneously, storing and releasing energy with changes in body motion.

So what happens when a rubber cord gets knots tied in it? The rubber cord's ability to store and release energy is immediately diminished. The same thing happens to your soft tissues when you build up restrictions and adhesions (from the micro-tears caused by repetitive motion), or scar tissue from injuries. These adhesions and scar tissues are analogous to knots in the cord. Just as the cord's ability to store and release energy was diminished by knots, so is our body's ability to store and release energy diminished by these restrictions. Think of these adhesions and restrictions as *energy leaks* that rob your body of much needed energy for healing.

You will have problems with storing and releasing your own energy if your body is full of tight areas and ropy fibrous restrictions.This is why foam rollers, Massage Therapy, Active Release Techniques, Graston Techniques, and dozens of other soft tissue techniques are so valuable for helping in your healing process. All these procedures act to improve the quality of your soft tissue by releasing or removing the soft tissue restrictions that lie between your tissue layers.

Bottom line: you may need to invest in some soft tissue care to get rid of these restrictions...these restrictions are sapping your energy, causing injuries, and aging you prematurely. Consider getting treatment for these areas. Obtaining care in this area is an investment that will pay countless positive dividends to you for the rest of your life.

Principle 3: Build your Aerobic Base

Yes, rehabilitative care does require you to build a good aerobic base. Your cardiovascular system is responsible for transporting oxygen and nutrients to all your cells, and for carrying away toxins and waste products. These are essential processes for any kind of recovery from injuries, and even more essential if you plan to take up athletic endeavours.

See the following topics for more information about the importance of Aerobic warm-ups:

Athletic or Performance Care Routines

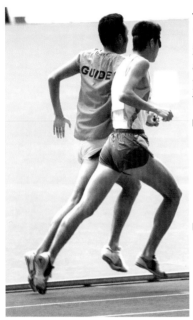

The major focus of the *Release Your Kinetic Chain* series of books is to help you resolve your injuries and to prepare your body for possible performance-level training.

- If your primary objective is to resolve an injury and you have no interest in athletic or performance care, then you can move directly to the next chapter.

- For the rest of you, there are several factors you should consider once you have attained a level of fitness where your body is ready to begin performance training.

Athletic performance training is all about speed, power, and strength, which in turn are based on the development of superb neuromuscular control. Great neuromuscular control (the training of your nervous system to perform a task) is what defines the world's best athletes – not strength or muscle size. There are some similarities (as well as some huge differences) in the objectives of rehabilitative exercise and athletic or performance training. In both, the development of neuromuscular control remains critical.

Athletic or Performance training has greater risks than rehabilitation training. Athletic training often involves riding the fence between overloading the body (to increase strength and power) and reaching the point of tissue failure (injury). In Performance training there is always a greater chance of injury. Athletic or performance training differs from rehabilitative training in its:

- Increased risk of injury.
- Need to work through muscle pain.

- Need to increase resistance to the point of overloading the muscles.
- Requiring speed training.
- Development of the anaerobic system.

The following are a few fundamental principles that you should keep in mind as you progress into Athletic training routines:

- *Principle 1: Athletic Development is Not the Same as Body-Building! - page 11*

- *Principle 2: Good Tissue Quality = Good Performance - page 12*

- *Principle 3: Some Muscle Pain is Okay - page 13*

- *Principle 4: Develop Your Aerobic Zone Before Working on Your Anaerobic Zone - page 14*

Principle 1: Athletic Development is Not the Same as Body-Building!

Exercise programs that focus only on increasing muscle size serve to meet *body-building* objectives of increasing size and definition and have very little to do with improved athletic performance or improved body function.

Athletic Performance training typically focuses upon developing your speed, power, and strength. To achieve this goal, you must establish good muscle endurance, good motor control, and superb neuromuscular responses. This is very different from body-building which focuses primarily on increasing the size and bulk of your muscles.

Exercise programs that focus only on increasing muscle size by isolating specific muscles (weight training with machines) often result in muscular imbalances, soft tissue injuries, and an overall decrease in performance. This is one of the reasons we do not recommend the use of exercise machines (other than cable machines) in any of our routines.

Look for athletic training programs that integrate elements of strength, endurance, speed, and power. These are the ones that will be most helpful in increasing your performance.

Principle 2: Good Tissue Quality = Good Performance

In sports performance, the quality of your soft tissue is a key element that cannot be ignored. When you improve the quality of your tissue (no restrictions, adhesions, or tightness) then you will reap the rewards of faster recovery, increased speed, improved range of motion, more strength, reduced injuries, and improved performance.

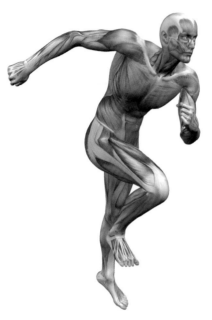

As we discussed in *Principle 2: Develop your Power - page 7,* your muscles are like rubber bands. When there are no knots (restrictions) in them you can easily store and release your energy. This directly translates into improved performance. This is why soft tissue techniques such as Active Release Techniques have helped take Olympic athletes to gold medal status. These types of techniques work to improve the overall quality of your soft tissues.

Bottom line: When you ignore the quality and state of your soft tissues, then you are taking the path of diminished performance! So, if you have restrictions and tight spots that are not resolved by exercising, then take the time to work these restrictions out by using our myofascial techniques (foam rollers, golf balls, self-massage) or see a skilled soft tissue practitioner for help in restoring your soft tissue quality. See *Alternative Therapies to Explore - page 221* for more information.

Principle 3: Some Muscle Pain is Okay

With performance training, it is often necessary to work through your muscle pain.

I am often asked the question, *"How do I know the difference between acceptable muscle pain and injury pain?"*

Muscle pain from exercising will usually diminish with time, but pain from an injury will not. I tell my patients that they should never work an area if they feel constant pain even when they are *not* exercising.

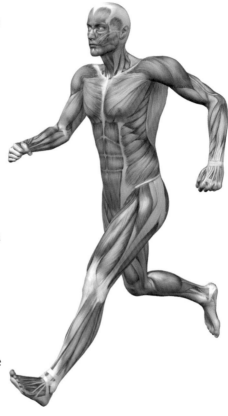

Pain from an injury is usually quite distinctive with sharp, stabbing sensations – or much more intense than normal muscle pain. It is also common to have injury-related pain increase with physical activity.

If you are injured, you need to return to a rehabilitative approach in your exercise program (for the affected structure). Working through injury-related pain is a sure way of continuing the injury or creating even more severe problems.

Principle 4: Develop Your Aerobic Zone Before Working on Your Anaerobic Zone

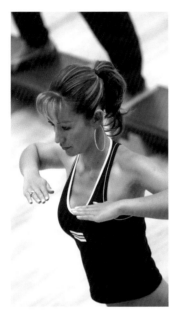

Anaerobic training (in which your tissues are working with reduced oxygen levels) is an essential aspect of performance training. However, as we mentioned earlier, you must first establish a good aerobic base before you can even consider beginning your anaerobic training.

Athletes who fail to train their aerobic base to a sufficient level before embarking on anaerobic training (intervals) can find themselves dealing with soft tissue injuries, diminished energy, slow healing, and even decreased performance levels. See *Working within your Aerobic and Anaerobic Zones - page 20* for more details about aerobic training.

The anaerobic or lactate system is very different from your aerobic system since it only operates for 5 seconds to about 2 minutes at a time. This anaerobic system is very efficient at producing power, but it also produces a considerable amount of waste by-products.

Do not start anaerobic training until you have established and maintained your *aerobic base* for several months. Once you start anaerobic training, your *Lactate Threshold* is established as you move back and forth between your aerobic and anaerobic systems. Your goal is to increase your anaerobic capacity (Lactate Threshold) since this will allow you to train for longer periods of time (within your aerobic zone), at faster speeds, and with greater intensity. A higher Lactate Threshold will also allow you to recover faster from your workouts.

Comparing the Benefits of Aerobic and Anaerobic Training

Cardiovascular warm-ups are all about increasing your circulatory function and increasing your energy production. Building up your aerobic base makes you heal faster, perform better, and even turns back your biological clock! Aerobic exercise does this by:

■ Increasing the density of capillaries in your muscles.

■ Increasing the mitochondrial function of your cells

Serious anaerobic training should only be taken up after you have built a good aerobic base. Anaerobic training causes your body to increase its production of Human Growth Hormone, which brings a whole host of health benefits to your body.

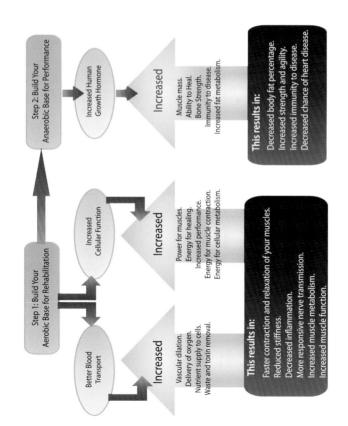

Step 1: Build Your Aerobic Base for Rehabilitation

Step 2: Build Your Anaerobic Base for Performance

Better Blood Transport

Increased Cellular Function

Increased Human Growth Hormone

Increased

Vascular dilation.
Delivery of oxygen.
Nutrient supply to cells.
Waste and toxin removal.

Increased

Power for muscles.
Energy for healing.
Increased performance.
Energy for muscle contraction.
Energy for cellular metabolism.

Increased

Muscle mass.
Ability to Heal.
Bone Strength.
Immunity to disease.
Increased fat metabolism.

This results in:

Faster contraction and relaxation of your muscles.
Reduced stiffness.
Decreased inflammation.
More responsive nerve transmission.
Increased muscle metabolism.
Increased muscle function.

This results in:

Decreased body fat percentage.
Increased strength and agility.
Increased immunity to disease.
Decreased chance of heart disease.

What is the Importance of Aerobic Warm-ups?

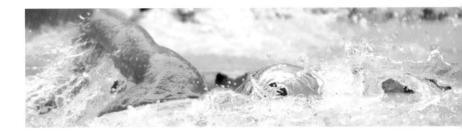

It may sound a little strange when we tell you to "warm up" your entire body, especially when you feel that your pain is localized in one area like your jaw, neck, or shoulder, and you just want to get started on resolving that particular issue.

But this initial aerobic workout (lasting for 10 to15 minutes) is one of the *first* things you should do before you ever begin working on your injured or restricted areas, and definitely before you begin any exercise routine.

What Happens During Aerobic Warm-ups

The aerobic warm-up helps to prepare your body, both physically and mentally, for the upcoming exercises by:

- Increasing circulation to your tissues.
- Preparing your heart for the upcoming exertions.
- Warming your tissues and thereby reducing your chances of injury.
- Making your muscles more flexible and ready for action.
- Priming and preparing your nervous system for new instructions.
- Improving your reaction times.
- Speeding healing of existing injuries.
- Increasing the mitochondrial function of your cells.

Improving Cellular Function with Aerobic Exercises

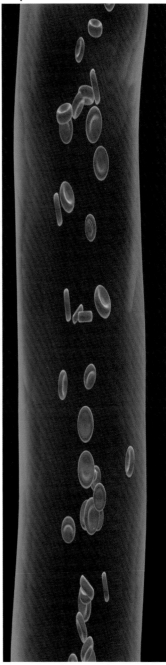

Aerobic exercise is the fastest way to increase the strength and function of your cardiovascular system. By increasing the density of capillaries, you are able to get more nutrients into your muscular tissue, thereby helping them to heal and perform better.

The increased density of capillaries means that you are better able to eliminate the waste by-products of healing and metabolism from your cells, again allowing them to perform more efficiently.

Aerobic exercise also increases the function of mitochondria in your cells. This increased mitochondrial function immediately boosts your body's ability to generate power and energy since your mitochondria are the principal energy generators for your cells.

Mitochondria convert existing nutrients into ATP (adenosine triphosphate), a form of energy that is readily usable by all the cells in your body. Your body uses this energy to perform all of its functions – from healing existing injuries, to eliminating waste, to powering your muscles when you walk, talk, or perform any action.

As we age, or when we injure ourselves, our ability to produce ATP decreases. Exercise is one of the few factors that will naturally increase ATP production to give you increased energy.

Aerobic Warm-Ups...how they helped resolve my injury!

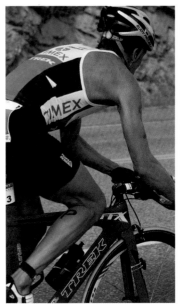

I have had a personal experience that showed me the importance of cardiovascular warm-ups as they relate to recovering from an injury.

I am speaking about an injury for which most people would never perform an aerobic workout. A few years ago I suffered from a severe case of *Bell's Palsy* (weakness of the nerve that innervates and controls the muscles for facial expression) on one-half of the face.

Bell's Palsy left me with the muscles of one-half of my face paralyzed and expressionless. I was told it would take 3 to 6 months before normal nerve function would be restored!

I was unwilling to live with this condition for that long and immediately researched means for reducing this time frame. One of the first things I did after getting Bell's Palsy was to get on my road bike/wind trainer for at least 20 to 30 minutes each day. I followed this up with TMJ massage and a variety of jaw, neck, and shoulder exercises.

To everyone's amazement, I recovered fully, with complete neuromuscular control of the muscles in my face, within about a month. I am convinced that my daily aerobic exercise is one of the major reasons I got over this condition in about a third of the normal time. The aerobic exercises I did every day resulted in increased circulatory function and improved mitochondrial activity (energy production)!

So take the time to do your aerobic warm-up before doing these exercise programs...you will be amazed at the difference it makes in your healing, recovery, power, and strength development!

So What is a Good Warm-up?

A good warm-up should include all the large muscles of your body and include movements that increase your heart rate and breathing. This is a good opportunity to *listen* to your body, and recognize any injury, tight spots, or restrictions that you may have to accommodate during your exercise routine.

- **Go for a brisk 10–to–20 minute walk.** Make sure you move your shoulders and swing your arms. Good upper extremity motion takes the stress off your back and helps you to store and release energy from your core. Don't walk at a slow pace, this will not achieve the desired results and is actually quite hard on your back compared to brisk walking.

- **Jog, or run for 10 to 20 minutes.** If you are not a runner, start with a brisk walk interspersed with a few short jogs. If you are a runner, make sure you maintain a good upright posture with good shoulder movement, and make sure you land on the middle of your feet. No toe or heel running as this deactivates your gluteals and causes a lot of other problems. Treadmills are fine but do not increase your elevation too much.

- **Swim for 20 minutes.** If you are doing the front crawl, make sure you breathe from both sides. You don't want your warm-up to create neuromuscular imbalances because you breathe from just one side of your body.

- **Use an elliptical or ski machine for 10 to 20 minutes.** Both are good for reinforcing a cross-crawling pattern, which helps establish good neuromuscular control, as well as for warming up all the big muscles of your body.

- **Ride a stationary bike for 10 to 20 minutes.** This option is not my first choice due to the lack of motion in the upper extremity. In terms of bike types, I prefer the use of upright bikes much more since you can maintain better posture, especially if you have a history of back pain.

- **Hula-hoop for 5 to 10 minutes.** Most people may not think of this as an aerobic exercise, but it is! The hula-hoop is not only a lot of fun, but it is also a great way to learn how to properly brace your core – a key concept in core stability.

Working within your Aerobic and Anaerobic Zones

Your warm-up, like all initial aerobic activity, needs to be performed within your aerobic zone. This is the range within which you want your heart to operate while you are performing your aerobic exercise. Think of your aerobic zone as the base which you must first establish for rehabilitation, and also for moving into the higher levels of performance in your chosen activity.

Calculating your aerobic zone - Use the following formula to calculate your *aerobic zone*:

1. Subtract your age from the number **220**.
   - For example, if I am **40** years old, then **220 - 40 = 180**.
2. Obtain the low end of your aerobic range by multiplying the result of step 1 by **0.6**.
   - In our example: **180 * 0.6 = 108**
3. Obtain the high end of your aerobic range by multiplying the result of step 1 by **0.7**.
   - In our example: **180 * 0.7 = 126**

This is your *aerobic heart rate zone* within which you need to work to develop your aerobic capacity. It is the zone which will best speed your recovery from an injury. If you work above this zone you run the risk of injury. If you work below this zone, you will not achieve the maximum benefits provided by your aerobic warm-up.

Calculating your anaerobic zone - Calculate the ideal heart-rate for your *anaerobic zone* by using the following procedure:

1. Subtract your age from the number **220**.
   - For example, if I am **40** years old, then **220 - 40 = 180**.
2. Obtain the low end of your anaerobic range by multiplying the result of step 1 by **0.8**.
   - In our example: **180 * 0.8 = 144**
3. Obtain the high end of your anaerobic range by multiplying the result of step 1 by **0.85**.
   - In our example: **180 * 0.85 = 153**

This is your *anaerobic heart rate zone* within which you need to work to develop your anaerobic capacity. It is the zone which will best assist in increasing muscle mass, speed healing, and increase immunity to disease.

Interval Training and Anaerobic Zones -

Interval training is the classic method for increasing your anaerobic zone. There are many books, references, and sports specialists who can help coach you through this process.

Find a good program that works for you and keep the following tips in mind as you start interval training:

- Before doing any type of interval training, always warm up for at least 10 to 15 minutes within your easy or low aerobic zone.
- Train within your anaerobic range for a maximum of 3 minutes.
- Then return to your 0.6 to 0.7 (aerobic) level for five to seven minutes. Your heart rate should return to this 60%- 70% range when you are doing your aerobic training. If it does not, consider this to be an indication that you need to spend more time developing your aerobic capacity.

Note: I highly recommend purchasing a heart rate monitor if you are going to work on increasing your aerobic capacity. They are well worth the investment.

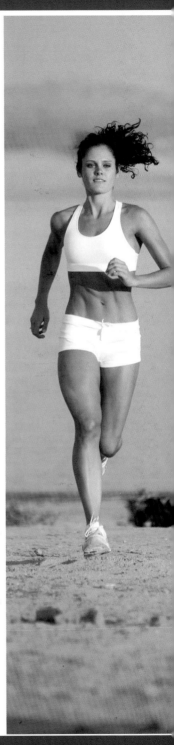

Involving Your Core

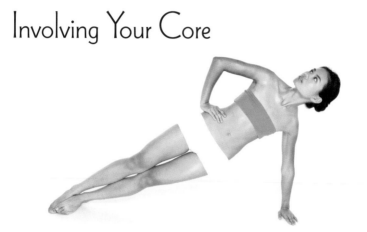

It doesn't matter what type of exercise you are performing; all exercises require good posture and solid support from your core. Your core is the foundation and source of all your movements, providing a stable base for all arm, leg, and neck motions. Your ability to maintain good posture is greatly dependent upon your core stability!

If you have a stable, balanced, elastic core, then you can easily transfer energy from the centre of your body to all your extremities! This process of first storing energy, and then releasing it, is very similar to how a spring mechanism works. A compressed spring contains stored energy. When the spring releases, the stored energy is released to allow the spring to expand. The muscles of your core act like a spring, compressing or tightening to store energy, and expanding to release the stored energy for use in movement!

Having the ability to store and release energy from your core is a fundamental aspect of injury resolution and athletic performance. It does not matter how fit you currently are, what your age is, or what your current health status is...you can always improve the quality of your core.

If you do not have a strong core, you rob yourself of much needed power and energy, and make yourself more susceptible to injuries.

Bracing Your Core

Almost all of our exercises require you to activate, brace, and otherwise involve your core! One of the key ways that all exercises can be converted into *core* exercises is through the process of **bracing**. I first learned about this process from Dr. Stuart McGill, Department Chair of the Spine Biomechanics Laboratory at the University of Waterloo.

Bracing refers to the process of *"contracting all the muscles in the abdominal wall without drawing or pushing in"*[1]. This is very different from the common advice given by some trainers to suck in (or hollow-out) your abdominals or to contract (pull in) your Transversus Abdominis muscle (TVA). In fact, Dr. McGill's research has shown that the action of *pulling in* your TVA actually **de-activates your paraspinal muscles** causing increased instability by creating or reinforcing abnormal neuromuscular patterns.

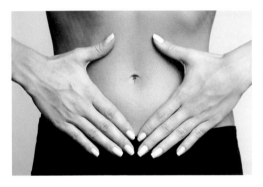

Basically, bracing is the process of gently pushing out while contracting all of your abdominal muscles.

This process also forces your paraspinal muscles to tighten at the same time.

The process of bracing creates a belt or corset around the core of your body which gives you a base of stabilization. This base of stability allows you to direct energy from your core to your extremities.

---

1. Ultimate Back Fitness and Performance, 3rd Edition, Stuart McGill PhD. 2004, Wabuno Publishers, BackFitPro Publishers.

How to Brace your Core!

Bracing is accomplished by gently pushing *out* your abdominal wall while tightening your back at the same time. This is actually quite a simple procedure once you get used to it. When bracing is is done correctly, you will almost immediately feel like you have a stronger core.

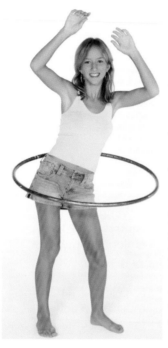

Another way to quickly learn how to brace is by using a hula-hoop.

That's right...your childhood toy can help you brace properly, especially when you use a weighted hula-hoop. Hula-hooping forces you to brace all your abdominal and back muscles at the same time.

Many adults are surprised to discover just how difficult hooping can be initially, especially when their children find it to be so easy. This is because children generally have better core strength than their parents.

Just five minutes of hula-hooping a day can substantially increase your core stability.

Note: For a better understanding of your core, I recommend reading Dr. Stuart McGill's book, "**Ultimate Back Fitness and Performance**".

Activating Your Hips

Seeing as we are on the topic of core stability, you also need to think about another key area of your core...your *hips*! A great deal of your core stability actually comes from your hips... an essential part of your kinetic chain and certainly not the part of your body that most of us would associate with dysfunctions and problems in your extremities (neck, shoulders, arms, hands, legs, feet, etc.).

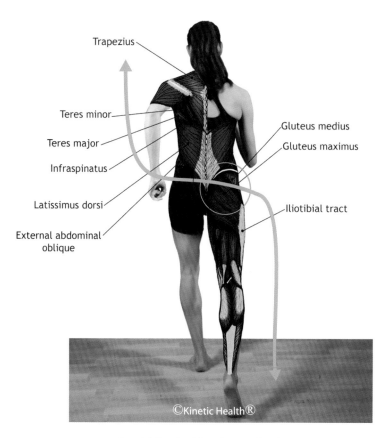

A restriction in either the muscles that surround the hip, or the hip capsule could affect the function of the upper and lower extremities.

Your hips also act as shock absorbers when you walk, run, or perform any action involving your legs. When your hip capsules and the muscles surrounding them move easily and freely, your body is able to store and release the force/energy generated when your feet strike the ground.

In contrast, a lack of hip motion (due to restrictions in either the hip capsule or the hip muscles) will often cause excessive force to be directed into the lower back and knees. This lack of force dissipation results in your body making compensations from your lower back into your neck and shoulders and can cause a series of chronic injuries.

This type of compensation is often seen in golfers who suffer from chronic shoulder injuries due to a lack of hip motion. Every time the golfer swings, he or she has to over-compensate for their restricted hip with excessive rotation of their shoulders. This usually results in neck, shoulder, and sometimes even jaw pain! Sound familiar?

Another major problem that occurs in conjunction with hip restriction is osteoarthritis. Restrictions in your hip prevent proper dissipation of force. Ideally this energy is stored and released with normal leg motion. However if, due to restrictions, the head of your femur (leg bone) is jamming directly into your pelvis (socket joint), you will see excessive wear and tear of the hip joint. This eventually leads to osteoarthritis, and in some cases, to a preventable hip replacement.

Basically if your hips are restricted, your body will compensate for this lack of motion by creating excessive motion in other parts of your body. Stress in your low back (due to lack of hip motion) causes compensations all the way back up to your shoulders and your neck.

The key point is that hip restrictions are often a contributing factor for many injuries which are distant from that area.

Testing your Core Stability - So let's do a simple test to see just how stable your core is currently! Professor Vladimir Janda – a neurologist specializing in manual medicine, and Dr. Craig Liebenson[1] first showed me variations of this test several years ago. Since then, well known author – Mark Verstegen – has added some very important refinements. And don't be upset if you fail; many top athletes fail this too!

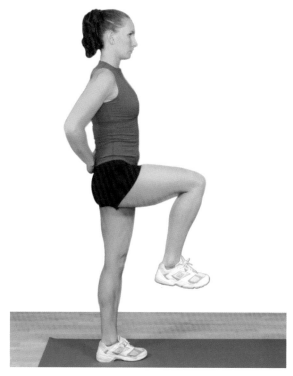

1. Starting Position:
    - Stand with good posture, next to a wall and in front of a mirror.
    - Centre your weight so that both feet are evenly balanced.
2. Lift one leg up, bending at the knee, to 90 degrees.
    - Keep your back and supporting leg straight.
3. Now flex your foot to 90 degrees and hold this position for about 30 to60 seconds.
    - If you have trouble with balance (cannot hold this position) then your core is unstable or unbalanced.

---

1. Craig Liebenson, Editor 1996, *Rehabilitation of the Spine: A Practitioner's Manual*,

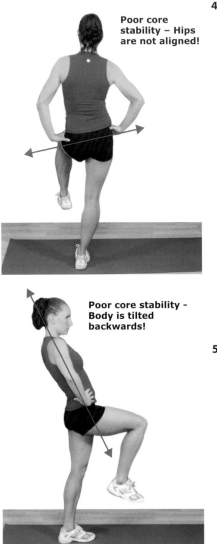

Poor core stability – Hips are not aligned!

Poor core stability - Body is tilted backwards!

4. Take a look at your hips:
   - Are both hips even or is one hip lower than the other?
   - If you are not able to maintain balanced hips, then your core is not stable.
   - If you are not able to even out your hips, you are probably not activating your gluteal muscles effectively.

   This indicates that you are transferring a lot of stress to your back and shoulders, which causes the structures of the upper extremity to over-compensate, leading to injuries.

5. Finally, are you able to maintain your balance without leaning forward or back?
   - If you have to compensate to maintain your balance, then your core is not stable.
   - Lack of core stability decreases your ability to transfer power to your arms, and leads to injuries of the upper extremity.

For more information, we recommend reading "Core Performance"[1] by Mark Verstegen. This book is an excellent source of information for improving your athletic performance.

---

1.   Core Performance Endurance, Mark Verstegen and Pete Williams. 2007 by JOXY LLC. Rodale Inc.

Balancing Flexibility with Control

Flexibility describes the range of movement possible in a joint or series of joints. You may be very flexible through certain joints, and remain quite inflexible in others. Regular stretching exercises can help to increase your range of motion (ROM)...but stretching should not be overdone!

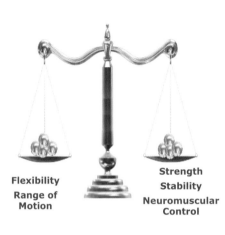

Flexibility
Range of
Motion

Strength
Stability
Neuromuscular
Control

Good flexibility is very important and is a key aspect of all our exercise routines, but flexibility alone is not enough to decrease your potential for injury.

In many cases, too much flexibility training can actually lead to injuries, especially if it is not balanced with strength, stability, and good neuromuscular control.

There is a fundamental rule you should follow when it comes to stretching. *You should only stretch a muscle to the length necessary to perform your selected task or sport.* For example, if you are a runner, you only want to improve or increase your flexibility to the point required by your stride length. Increasing your flexibility past this point makes no sense since it can cause decreased power availability (like an overstretched spring), cause instability, increase your chances of injury, and perhaps even decrease your overall performance.

Some people are incredibly flexible, and still suffer from musculoskeletal pain. This is because their hyper-mobile or loose joints are very unstable and easily injured. Great flexibility through your joints is meaningless without good stability.

One of the key reasons that you should stretch is to correct imbalances in specific muscle groups. For example, when one of your hamstrings is much less flexible than the other, the resulting imbalance can easily lead to injury. It is often more important to correct this asymmetry than it is to aim for an overall increase in range of motion. In other words, you want to achieve a state where both hamstrings have equal flexibility, and can work together in a balanced and coordinated manner.

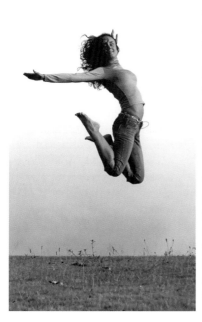

As we discussed earlier, force generation in your body is a process of *storage* and *release*. Your body is just like a spring, which stores energy in its compressed form, and releases it when uncompressed.

If you unwind your muscular spring mechanism too much (by over-stretching), then you substantially diminish the amount of energy or power that these muscles can generate.

Your goal is to achieve a balance (or symmetry) in your flexibility, to obtain sufficient range of motion for performing the action you require for your sport or activity, while continuing to maintain the power of the spring mechanism in your muscles.

Important areas in which you typically need to develop good symmetrical range of motion include your jaw, neck, shoulders, core, hips, knees, and ankles.

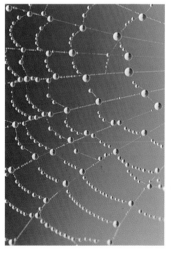

Shoulder to Hand - a Kinetic Chain

Shoulder, elbow, wrist, and *hand*...what's the connection? We don't normally think of the interconnections between these structures until we suffer from pain or injury to them. However, when we are unable to perform our activities of daily living, we become all too aware of these inter-relationships. Without properly functioning muscles, tendons, ligaments, joints, and connective tissue from your shoulders to your hands, you would find yourself unable to perform many of the complex daily tasks that are required by your job and home life.

What is a Kinetic Chain?

The structural inter-dependencies between the muscles, tendons, ligaments, joints, and fascia of your body comprises a **Kinetic Chain**.

You can think of your body as being comprised of a series of small kinetic chains, each linked to other kinetic chains to form a complex body-encompassing **Kinetic Web**! Tension or injury to any part of this kinetic chain would affect the function of all its linked components.

Visualizing the Kinetic Chain

You can visualize the kinetic chain from your shoulder to hand as a layered, multi-level spider web. In your body, this web is made up of soft-tissue fibres (muscles, tendons, ligaments, and connective tissue). In some areas where are there are multiple *layers* of muscle and soft tissue, this complex web can be seven-or-eight layers thick. Like all natural webs, each kinetic web is unique to each individual's unique anatomy, and can vary structurally depending on that person's environmental and genetic factors.

Just like a spider's web, if you were to pull or increase tension in one of the fibres, this tension would resonate throughout the entire web. However, unlike the two-dimensional spiderweb, this resonance would be felt *above, below, beside*, and *behind* the affected fibre. Thus, damage to muscle fibres in one area would affect the function of tissues in multiple layers, through multiple planes of motion, and at multiple locations.

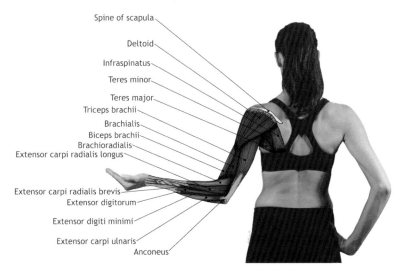

Spine of scapula
Deltoid
Infraspinatus
Teres minor
Teres major
Triceps brachii
Brachialis
Biceps brachii
Brachioradialis
Extensor carpi radialis longus
Extensor carpi radialis brevis
Extensor digitorum
Extensor digiti minimi
Extensor carpi ulnaris
Anconeus

Unfortunately, the majority of medical schools do not teach anatomy with these interconnections in mind. Sadly, anatomy is usually taught as if each separate structure was floating in space, with little or no emphasis on the effects of that structure's interconnections to its surrounding tissues. A better way to learn anatomy would be to understand how each structure's fibres *connects into the next structure,* and how each component of our musculoskeletal system *affects the function* of every other structure.

When a muscle contracts, many other muscles also contract (or relax) in different directions, gliding over each other. All of these actions are supported by the core of your body and directed by your nervous system. This synergistic dance of complexity is truly amazing!

Shoulder to Arm - A Kinetic Chain

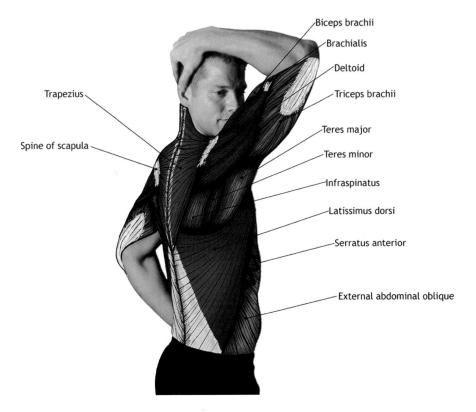

Biceps brachii
Brachialis
Deltoid
Triceps brachii
Teres major
Teres minor
Infraspinatus
Latissimus dorsi
Serratus anterior
External abdominal oblique

Trapezius
Spine of scapula

Most shoulder and arm problems occur due to muscle imbalances, adhesion formation between soft tissues, and a lack of neuromuscular control. These problems often involve the numerous osseous (bone) and soft tissue structures that extend

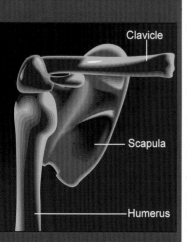

Clavicle

Scapula

Humerus

The following are some of the muscles that attach to the shoulder blade (scapula).

- Biceps Brachii (short and long head)
- Coracobrachialis
- Deltoid
- Infraspinatus
- Latissimus Dorsi (some fibres)
- Levator Scapulae
- Pectoralis Minor
- Rhomboid Major
- Rhomboid Minor
- Serratus Anterior
- Subscapularis
- Supraspinatus
- Teres Major
- Teres Minor
- Trapezius

from your lower extremity, through your core, and out into your extremities.

Shoulder movement is a highly synergistic activity that requires precise coordination. Consider some of the intricacy in the shoulder complex, with accompanying stabilization by the core of your body.

The shoulder complex is made of three bones: shoulder blade (scapula), collar bone (clavicle), and the upper arm (humerus). In addition, three joints play important roles in shoulder movement:

- **The Glenohumeral** joint occurs where the upper arm (humerus) inserts into the socket on the end of the shoulder blade (glenoid fossa) and is surrounded by a ligamentous capsule.

- The second joint is the **Sternoclavicular** (SC) joint which allows movement to occur between the collar bone (clavicle) and the breastbone (sternum).

- The third joint, the **Acromioclavicular** (AC) joint allows movement to take place between the outer collar bone (clavicle) and the acromion process of the shoulder blade (scapula).

Multiple muscles attach to each of these three bones and are involved in specific shoulder actions (protraction, retraction, rotation, etc). A restriction in just one of these muscles can affect the function of the entire shoulder complex, and result in Scapular Dyskinesis (abnormal shoulder motion).

Numerous studies have shown how an alteration in normal shoulder blade motion can lead to several shoulder injuries and shoulder impingement syndromes.

Core Stability and Your Shoulder

Core stability plays a key kinetic chain role in the rehabilitation of any shoulder injury or when attempting to improve athletic performance. The muscles of the core stabilize the spine and form the base from which power is generated and distributed to the shoulders and arms.

All forceful actions are initiated from the centre of the body and are expressed outward. When you don't have a strong, stable, balanced core, you will find that your body continually wastes energy with each action that you perform.

I like the analogy that Paul Chek[2] (C.H.E.K. Institute) uses when describing the importance of core function and stability. Paul talks about how a golf swing without core stability is much the same as shooting a cannon from a row boat. Obviously, without a solid base or foundation for the cannon, there is little or no control on where the cannon ball lands. The same concept applies to all shoulder-arm actions! The results of injury rehabilitation or sport performance training are very limited when one has poor core stability.

Case Study - Golf and Your Kinetic Chain

To get a better understanding of the core–torso–shoulder–arm kinetic chain relationship, I would like to share a story about one of our patients, Michelle (*not her real name*), an avid golfer who is on the golf course every chance she gets.

Due to its high injury rates, Golf provides us with many opportunities for demonstrating kinetic chain relationships. Up to 60% of golfers are injured each year, with an even higher number of injuries occurring in the senior population. Often these injuries are

2. The Golf Biomechanics Manual, Whole in One Golf Conditioning. Paul Chek. 1999, A C.H.E.K Institute Publication.

a result of lack of physical conditioning or are due to compensations for existing soft-tissue restrictions. Golf is definitely not a low-impact sport!

Michelle was first referred to our clinic (Kinetic Health, Calgary) with a case of Golfers Elbow (Medial Epicondylitis) along with chronic rotator cuff problems. Michelle also had secondary complaints of chronic low back pain and right anterior rib pain, which on occasion could be very severe. Michelle had already seen several different types of practitioners for her complaints, but had not seen a resolution to her problems.

First, we ran Michelle through the normal orthopedic and neurological tests. The most predominant findings were the hypertonic muscles in her shoulders, elbows, low back, and along her ribs. Functional examinations also showed several imbalances in her core stability (weak hips and balance issues).

We then performed a video analysis of her golf swing. A typical golf swing can be divided into several biomechanical phases: *Address Position, Takeaway, Forward Swing, Acceleration, Follow-Through* and *Late Follow-Through.*

Through each phase, we focused our analysis upon our patient's ability to perform the motion, with the correct body sequence, smoothly and efficiently. In addition, we paid attention to the sequential and kinetic transfer of power (*Kinematic Sequence)* through the body. Ideally we should first see motion in the golfer's hips, generating the power which is transferred through the torso, into the arms, and finally down the club and into the club head.

We always leave recommendations about the actual techniques involved in a golf swing to the Golf Pros. Instead, we focus upon *our* area of expertise – the identification of soft-tissue and joint restrictions, and the resolution of the neuromuscular problems caused by those restrictions – with an aim towards improving the patient's ability to perform the required actions.

In fact, we have found the *team approach* to be the most effective when attempting to improve an individual's golf swing. An ideal support team would consist of a Golf Pro, a Musculoskeletal Specialist (such as myself), an Exercise Trainer, and someone to help you with psychological and mental aspects of the game.

An efficient golf swing is a great example of power generation through the core. The twisting motion of your body during the golf swing produces an amazing amount of torque and rotational force. This force increases the velocity of the golf club head, with the resulting force being directed into the ball. The greater the speed of your club head, the more kinetic energy that is transferred to the golf ball.

Unfortunately, an inefficient golf swing still produces high levels of kinetic energy. However, instead of the energy being transferred into the golf ball, the kinetic energy is re-directed back into the soft tissues of your body. This results in micro-tears, which creates an inflammatory response, the formation of scar tissues, and a resultant decrease in mobility. With this in mind, let us review what we saw on Michelle's analysis.

An Analysis of Michelle's Kinetic Chain

Two important aspects of biomechanical analysis are the determination of the kinematic sequence and Electromyographic (EMG) analysis. Kinematic sequencing[3] of a golf swing shows how power is transferred from the hips and torso through the arms, and finally directed into the club head. Electromyographic[4] analysis[5] is used to determine which muscles are active through each phase of a golf swing. In Electromyography, electrodes are placed on the skin, and an instrument is used to measure the activity of the monitored muscles throughout the swing. This valuable information has shown clinicians which muscles are most active during each phase of the swing.

When an abnormal muscle-firing sequence or abnormal motion pattern is detected, the clinician can then look for a restriction or find weaknesses in the primary muscles involved in that phase of the swing[6]. The exact structures that are affected vary from individual to individual, and are dependent upon that person's anatomy, level of fitness, prior history of injuries, and the presence of existing physical restrictions.

---

3. Golf Workshop - Technique and 3D Biomechanics Workbook. Titleist Performance Institute. Acushnet Company 2006
4. Electromyographic Analysis of the Scapular Muscles During a Golf Swing, Am J Sports Med January 1995 vol. 23 no. 1 19-23
5. Feeling up to Par: Medicine from Tee to Green, Philadelphia, 1994: 9-13 McCaroll J.R., Mallon W.J., Epidemiology of Golf Injuries, In Stover C.N., McCaroll J.R., Mallon W.J.
6. Muscle activity during the golf swing, Br. J. Sports. Med. November 1, 2005 39:799-804 A McHardy, H Pollard, and P J Garbutt

We have found that combining information from kinematic sequencing, EMG studies, and our own video and biomechanical analysis works extremely well in improving the performance of even PGA and Nationwide Tour players. This biomechanical analysis give us great information about how a restriction or imbalance in one area of the body can cascade into multiple injuries in other parts of the body.

Address Phase - This is the initial starting position for a golf swing.

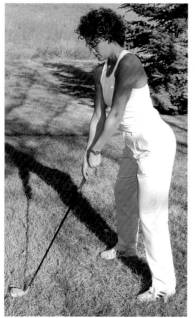

Model depicting the Address Phase of a golf swing.

With Michelle, during the initial address, we found that:

- Her shoulders were rolled forward - a common problem that greatly affects a golfer's power and distance. This is commonly known as a C-Posture, and is often caused by a combination of joint restrictions and muscle imbalances.

- Knee flexion was minimal and she had some difficultly maintaining the position (due to weak quadriceps) which affected her ability to maintain a proper spinal angle.

- Her ankles did not bend very much, especially on the right side (due to tight calf muscles) which affected her balance.

Takeaway Phase - Involves moving from the Address position into the Backswing Position. This phase is essentially a coiling of the upper body into a position where it can store energy for quick release. This is very similar to coiling up a spring, before releasing it. The lower body acts as the base from which the spring is released.

In general terms, a strong balanced core will protect your spine and promote good coil and recoil actions. This not only translates into a more powerful and accurate golf swing, but also serves to prevent a host of kinetic–chain–related injuries.

During the Takeaway phase:

- Some of the most active upper extremity muscles that play a critical role in stabilizing the upper body during the golf swing include the *Trapezius, Subscapularis, Levator Scapulae, Rhomboids, Supraspinatus, Infraspinatus and Pectoralis Major.*
- Some of the most active Core muscles that play an important role for a right-handed golfer are: *Gluteus Maximus, External Oblique (L), Internal Oblique (R), and the Erector Spinae (L).*

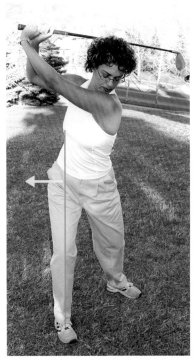

In addition to these muscles, the majority of golfers that we see at our clinic also have tight hip flexors (*Psoas/iliacus*). These hip flexors help to maintain a good spinal angle throughout the entire golf swing. Tight or restricted hip flexors commonly cause low back pain and a decrease in swing performance.

With Michelle, during the Takeaway phase, we found that:

- Hip motion was limited due to restrictions in hip muscles (especially her external hip rotators).
- Her entire spine had an anterior tilt, which greatly reduced her ability to generate power. With Michelle, this was partially due to tight hip flexors.
- She felt pain at the top of her backswing which is sometimes caused by an impingement syndrome.

Model depicting the Takeaway Phase of a golf swing, with a sway away from the target.

We also noticed that Michelle had a slight 'sway' during her Backswing. A 'Sway' refers to a lateral movement by the lower body *away* from the target during the back swing. This *sway* can be an indication of weak gluteal muscles, restricted hip rotation, or lack of joint mobility in the thoracic spine. Essentially Michelle had set the scene for multiple kinetic chain problems before she had even taken a swing at the ball.

Forward –Swing Phase - Involves moving from the Backswing, through the Down Swing, into the Horizontal Club position. During this phase, the right-handed golfer starts to uncoil the upper body while beginning to rotate the trunk in a counter-clockwise direction. The golfer shifts her weight to the left foot while at the same time her torso, hips, and knees turn synchronously to the left. This uncoiling motion occurs due to the contraction of the abdominal and paraspinal muscles.

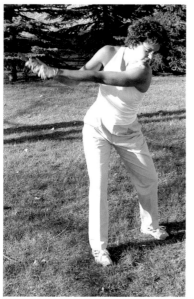

During the Forward-Swing phase:

- The lateral shoulder ligaments (*acromioclavicular ligaments*) are stretched.
- The shoulder blades (*scapulae*) are externally rotated.
- The three rotator cuff muscles (*subscapularis, infraspinatus,* and *teres minor*) work to stabilize the shoulder joint.
- The back muscles (*erector spinae*) stabilize the golfer's posture.
- The oblique abdominal muscles control the rotation and flexion of the torso.

Model depicting the Forward–Swing Phase of a golf swing.

The **Forward Swing** (and the **Acceleration Phase**) are the stages which create the greatest amount of spinal loading[7].The force exerted on a golfer's back during these actions is equivalent to eight times the golfer's body weight.[8] In contrast, runners only experience a force of three times their body weight, while rowers experience a force of seven times their body weight. This is an interesting finding when one considers that most people think of golf as being a low-impact sport. In fact, due to these forces, low-back pain is the golfers' most common complaint.

7. Electromyographic Analysis of the Scapular Muscles During a Golf Swing, Am J Sports Med January 1995 vol. 23 no. 1 19-23

8. Golf Injuries and Biomechanics of the Golf Swing, University of Umeå Department of Sports Medicine Sports Medicine, Katarina Grinell, Karin Henriksson-Larsén Gothenburg, January 25, 1999

During the **Downswing Phase**, the golfer's hips normally slide towards the target causing the lower back to tilt to the right. Too much of this side-bending action can be a major cause of low back pain.

With Michelle, during the **Forward Swing** phase, we found that she seemed to have a problem maintaining a smooth swing plane. In fact, her swing plane was very steep. A steep swing plane often pushes the hips laterally during the downswing, which in turn causes an increased hip slide on impact. Too much hip slide is often associated with an increase in low back pain.

Acceleration Phase - Involves moving from the Horizontal club position to ball contact. During this stage, muscle energy is converted into club head acceleration.

During the downswing, golfers often decelerate their swing just prior to hitting the ball. This deceleration places considerable stress on the common flexor tendon[9]. This is one reason why elbow injuries (Golfers Elbow) commonly occur at the point of ball impact. Poor strength and flexibility in the wrist, forearms and shoulder are other common reasons for elbow injuries.

During the Acceleration Phase of a right-handed golfer, some of the most active muscles are[10] :

- Upper extremity muscles are the *pectoralis* (most active during acceleration phase), *latissimus dorsi, trapezius, levator scapula,* and *rhomboids.*
- Core muscles are the left *gluteus maximus* (acts as a stabilizer at the time of ball impact), *external obliques, left internal oblique, erector spinae.*
- *Paraspinal* and *oblique abdominal muscles* become involved in core stabilization.
- *Oblique abdominals* become involved in the rotation of the trunk.

It is essential to maintain a balance between the forearm flexors and extensor. This balance allows for a good wrist-cock during the golf swing and acts to protect the hand and wrist during ball impact. With Michelle, during the Acceleration phase, we found that:

- She would slow down her swing just prior to making contact with the ball. As we mentioned earlier, this sudden deceleration is a very common cause of elbow injury.

---

9.   Stannish W.D., Loebenberg M.I., Kozey J.W., The Elbow, In Stover C.N., McCaroll J.R., Mallon W.J. Feeling up to Par: Medicine from Tee to Green, Philadelphia, 1994: 143-49
10. Golf Injuries and Biomechanics of the Golf Swing, University of Umeå, Department of Sports Medicine Sports Medicine, Katarina Grinell, Karin Henriksson-Larsén Gothenburg, January 25, 1999

■ She did not effectively shift her weight onto the leading side of her body. This lack of motion is often due to restrictions in the leading hip or a decrease in the strength of the tail leg.

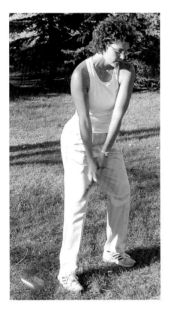

Due to Michelle's lack of flexibility and poor core strength, her body had to make numerous compensations in order to stay within the appropriate swing plane.

These compensations resulted in additional and considerable stress on her elbow.

Model depicting the Acceleration Phase of a golf swing.

Follow-Through Phase - Involves moving from ball contact to a horizontal club position. The Follow-Through phase begins with ball contact. During this phase your body rotates to the left with your spine acting as the central axis of rotation. In addition your hips and shoulders will rotate until your body is facing the target. 30% of all golfing injuries occur during the Follow-Through phase.

During the Follow-Through phase, several muscles work together to decelerate and control rotation through the use of eccentric muscle contractions. During an eccentric muscle contraction, the muscle produces force while it is actively lengthening. Eccentric muscle contractions are often used to control the speed of a movement by slowing down or decelerating a limb.[11]

In general, muscle activity decreases at this stage of the swing, with the exception of the left abdominal oblique muscle (for a right-handed golfer).

---

11. Golf Injuries and Biomechanics of the Golf Swing, University of Umeå, Department of Sports Medicine Sports Medicine, Katarina Grinell, Karin Henriksson-Larsén Gothenburg, January 25, 1999

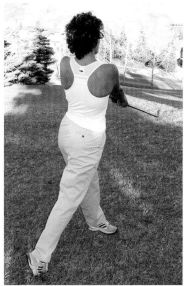

Model depicting the Follow Through-Phase of a golf swing.

During the Follow-Through Phase of a right-handed golfer:

- Some of the most active upper extremity muscles are the *latissimus dorsi, pectoralis major, right infraspinatus,* and *right subscapularis.*
- Some of the most active core muscles are the *gluteus maximus, external oblique, left internal oblique,* and the *erector spinae.* The gluteus muscles help to stabilize the pelvis and in conjunction with the latissimus Dorsi promotes rotation throughout the swing.

With Michelle, during the Follow-Through phase, we found that she lacked both spinal and hip rotation.

Late Follow-Through Phase - Involves moving from the horizontal club position to the final finish position. During this stage of the golf swing, trunk rotation is decelerating, and all muscle activity is decreasing with the exception of the left abdominal oblique (for the right-handed golfer).

During this phase your wrists rotate over each other to create the roll-over motion of your hands. Your spine hyper-extends, and your body weight fully shifts to the left side.

During the Late Follow-Through phase (for a right-handed golfer):

- Some of the most active upper extremity muscles are the *pectoralis major, infraspinatus,* and *subscapularis.*
- Some of the most active core muscles are the *gluteus maximus, external obliques, left internal oblique,* and *the erector spinae.*

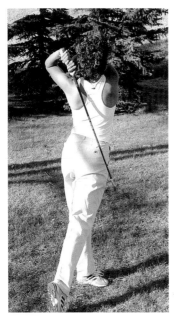

With Michelle, during the Late Follow-Through phase, we found that:

- Her lack of spinal and pelvic rotation was most evident during the end range of her Follow-Through phase.
- Her lower extremity appeared to be rather unstable during rotation. This was due to restrictions in muscles involved in lower extremity stabilization: the *peroneals, adductors, hamstrings* and *quadriceps.*

Model depicting the Late Follow-Through Phase of a golf swing.

Conclusion - Our biomechanical analysis of Michelle's golf swing revealed the following key factors:

- Michelle's lack of core stability, strength, and flexibility greatly altered her swing plane.
- The altered swing plane in combination with the deceleration in her swing before ball impact lead to, and perpetuated, her elbow problem.
- The repetitive motion of a golf swing created shoulder instability which eventually lead to shoulder impingement (pain on top of backswing).
- The chronic back pain was largely due to lack of core stability while performing high-velocity movements.

These factors greatly affected her *kinematic sequencing*[12], her ability to efficiently transfer force from her hip through her torso, into her shoulders and arms, and finally down to the head of her golf club.

Fortunately, we were able to help Michelle resolve all her biomechanical problems. Achieving this resolution required a good understanding of the key kinetic chain structures that were involved in her problem. By

---

12. Golf Workshop - Technique and 3D Biomechanics Workbook. Titleist Performance Institute. Acushnet Company 2006

following Michelle's kinetic chain links, we could see a pattern of dysfunction that ran from her upper extremity right down to her feet.

Even though Michelle's primary problem (area of most pain) appeared to be her elbow, the perpetuating factor was actually her shoulder (chronic rotator cuff injury). This chronic shoulder problem was caused by kinetic chain compensations for her body's lack of core stability and an over-compensation in her golf swing due to hip restrictions. Her lack of core stability was continually being exacerbated by a lack of stability in her lower extremities. Michelle's rib pain was also directly related to compensations generated by a weak and unstable core.

To resolve her problem, we applied a whole-body exercise program (similar to those in this book) in combination with soft tissue treatments such as Active Release Techniques and Massage. Within a relatively short time Michelle was back on the golf course, but without the chronic problems she faced before. And now she was able to execute the correct movements that her Swing Coach wanted.

This type of kinetic chain scenario occurs commonly with both sporting injuries and workplace injuries. As you can see from this case study, it is important to address the *entire* kinetic chain in order to resolve most chronic soft-tissue problems.

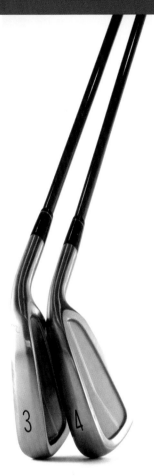

Becoming Aware of your Shoulder-to-Arm Kinetic Chain

It is very easy for you to learn how to become aware of your shoulder–to–arm kinetic chain and how this kinetic chain affects your ability to perform tasks! Lets take a look at a common upper extremity syndrome known as **Forward Shoulder Posture (FSP)**. FSP is common among office workers, students, and probably over half of the patients who walk through my front office doors.

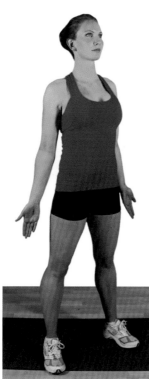

Anatomically Neutral Position

People with FSP exhibit rolled-forward shoulders, with a forward-tilted head, and raised shoulder blades. The onset of these postural changes is so slow and gradual that the majority of people don't even realize that they are exhibiting these postures when they sit or stand. In addition to these obvious postural changes, numerous mechanical changes also take place within their musculoskeletal and nervous systems.

Try the following test to experience just what happens to your wrist, elbow, hands, and neck with FSP!

1. **Starting Position**:
    Stand up with your shoulders back, arms by your side, and your palms facing for-ward.

    This is known as an Anatomically Neutral Position. In this position your thumbs will naturally point out to the side (externally rotated).

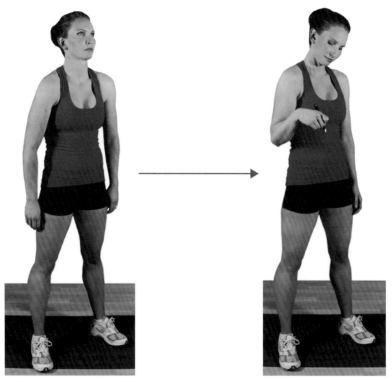

Forward Shoulder Posture

Testing the Kinetic Chain

2. **FSP Posture**: Now relax your arms and roll your shoulders as far forward as you can. This position causes your elbows and wrist to rotate inward (internally rotated), and your thumbs now point towards your body.

3. **Test Your Kinetic Chain**: Keeping your shoulders rotated forward, pretend that you are holding a pen and writing on an imaginary piece of paper. The first thing you will feel is the increased tension in your elbows, wrists, hands, and neck.

4. Now try performing some of your daily living tasks in this position!

Can you feel all the tension that would develop in all these areas? And can you see how much energy you waste by maintaining this energy–inefficient posture. Most people don't realize that poor posture not only causes injuries, but also saps your energy!

What you just experienced are some of the more obvious stresses placed on your kinetic chain by Forward Shoulder Posture. Unfortunately, most of the other changes that take place are not so obvious! The tension from FSP creates friction that results in micro-tears and adhesion formation in your muscles, ligaments, and tendons. These changes cause inflammation and the formation of scar tissue.

It often takes some time for these adhesions to build up to a point where they affect your ability to perform certain actions (which is usually when you notice them)! When you finally notice the problem, you may have no idea how it occurred! This is especially true if you experience these symptoms in your wrist or hand, but the actual problem is in your shoulder.

Even your nervous system can be affected without your being aware of it. Research has shown that FSP can actually cause tension and reduce normal motion (nerve sliding) of the Median nerve in your arm.[13] The Median nerve is most commonly associated with Carpal Tunnel Syndrome (CTS). Researchers have found that subjects who maintained an FSP posture developed Paresthesias – with abnormal sensations such as burning, tingling, or prickling.

These symptoms are commonly associated with Carpal Tunnel Syndrome, and many practitioners may then give patients exercises that *only* address the wrist, rather than using exercises that address the complete postural changes that caused FSP.

We have designed our exercise routines to address the needs of your kinetic chain, not just the symptomatic area. These routines will help you strengthen and heal, not just in the initial area of pain, but also all of the surrounding supportive soft tissues of that structure's kinetic chain.

13. Shoulder Posture and Median Nerve Sliding. Andrea Julius, Rebecca Lees, Andrew Dilley, Bruce Lynn BMC. Musculoskeletal Disorders. 2004:5:23. Published online 2004 July 28. doi:10.1186/1471-2474-5-23.

Nerve Entrapment in Your Arm

Nerve entrapment syndromes in the arm are more common than most people realize. These entrapment syndromes often occur as a result of repetitive strain injuries, previous traumas, poor posture, and de-conditioned muscles. Nerve entrapment can create major barriers during the rehabilitation of an injury or when attempting to improve sports performance.

When nerves are entrapped between tissue layers, your body will go to great lengths to protect these nerves by reducing muscle function. This results in muscle imbalances, abnormal neuromuscular responses, and a decreased ability to generate force.

Nerve entrapment syndromes typically involve both *motor* and *sensory* nerves. Entrapment of sensory nerves creates pain and paresthesias (sensations of tingling, pricking, increased sensitivity, or numbness). In such cases, sensory nerve entrapment is often obvious to the person.

Motor nerves allow the brain to stimulate muscle contraction. Entrapment of motor nerves causes weakness, decreased muscle function, and muscle atrophy (wasting away). In minor cases, the onset of motor nerve entrapment may be so slow and insidious that the person is never aware of his or her decrease in function.

To address nerve entrapment in the arm, we have included specific exercises to help release the entrapped nerves and restore function. These exercises are referred to as *nerve flossing* or *nerve gliding* exercises and they help to restore normal neuromuscular patterns, increase strength, and increase range of motion.

Basically a nerve flossing exercise is a procedure in which a nerve is minimally tensioned, while a specific motion is being performed. A common analogy compares flossing your teeth with nerve flossing. But in this case, the floss is your nerve, and instead of moving between your teeth, you are moving the nerve through soft tissue structures that may be entrapping that nerve.

Your Hand's Kinetic Chain

Your hands are amazing structures that (when fully functional) combine precise movements with strength and mobility. This requires all the joints, muscles, ligaments, tendons, connective tissue, and your nervous system to be fully coordinated and functional in their actions. This interplay of precision normally works extremely well until one of these anatomical links becomes damaged or restricted.

It is not always easy to know just which link has become dysfunctional. This is because many of the anatomical structures that control hand and wrist motion originate much farther up the arm and on the elbow. Consider the following two examples:

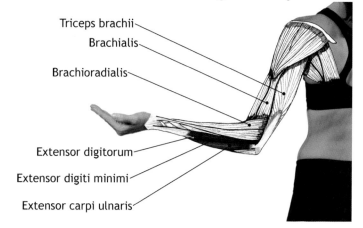

Triceps brachii
Brachialis
Brachioradialis

Extensor digitorum
Extensor digiti minimi
Extensor carpi ulnaris

■ *Extensor digitorum*: This muscle assists in the extension of your fingers (interphalangeal joints). Even though this muscle is involved in finger extension, it *originates* at the elbow (lateral epicondyle of the humerus). An injury to this muscle, or a restriction at the elbow, can directly affect finger movements.

■ *Extensor carpi ulnaris*: This muscle extends and moves the wrist towards the centre line (adducts). Again even though this muscle is involved in wrist motion, it originates on the outside of the elbow (*common extensor tendon*) and inserts into the wrist (at the base of the fifth metacarpal). An injury to this muscle near the elbow can directly affect wrist and hand motion.

Due to these anatomical relationships, any remedial exercise routines must include not just the structures involved in hand motion, but also other related structures that lie further up the arm, and sometimes even into the shoulder. In other words, the exercise routine must include all the related kinetic chain structures of the hand!

Thumb Motion

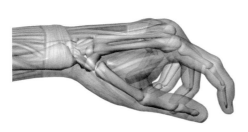

Hand injuries often involve problems with the thumb. Your thumb, unlike your other fingers, is an opposable digit, and is the only finger that is able to oppose or turn back against your other fingers.

This ability of the thumb (opposition) is the reason we are able to grip or hold objects, and is a key factor in our ability to perform our fine motor actions. In fact, it is hypothesized that much of our technological development would never have occurred without our opposable thumb.

Thumb opposition is a result of the combined actions of multiple joints and muscles moving in several directions. When thumb opposition is restricted, we must address several local structures including the *adductor pollicis, flexor pollicis brevis, opponens pollicis,* and *abductor pollicis brevis* which all attach into the thumb from either the wrist or hand.

In contrast, several thumb actions (extension, flexion, rotation) are controlled by muscles which originate further up the forearm. An example would be the following two structures:

- *Flexor pollicis longus,* which originates halfway up your forearm and is involved in the flexion of the thumb. Restrictions in this muscle affect your ability to flex the joints of your thumb.

- *Extensor pollicis brevis* which originates on the back of your forearm and is involved in the extension of the thumb. Restrictions in this muscle affect your ability to extend your thumb.

Bottom line, in order to resolve any hand injury, exercise and therapy must address not only the structures in the hand itself, but also include other structures that lie much farther up the hand's kinetic chain.

Applying Kinetic Chain Principles to Exercise

Our kinetic chain approach to resolving soft tissue injuries also applies to the exercise routines that we recommend for rehabilitating your soft tissues. You must always take into account the kinetic chain relationships of the structures that are injured!

The exercise routines in this book take into account the kinetic chain relationships of your shoulder, arm, and elbow. See the following chapters for some of the specific strengthening and stretching exercises that we recommend at our clinic for the prevention and treatment of arm, elbow, and shoulder injuries.

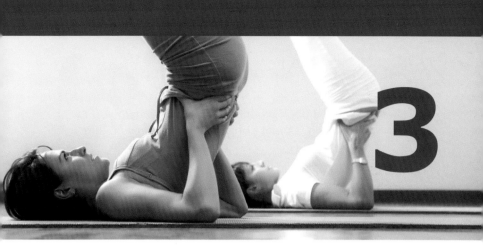

What's Special About These Exercises

Physical training is often poorly executed and misunderstood. All too often people become injured when they are asked to execute extremely challenging training programs without correct preparation of their body. Equally often, I see many athletes trying to work though the pain of their injury only to create a chronic, longer-lasting problem. This situation is usually the direct result of poorly-designed exercise programs.

This may sound strange, but many exercise programs contain components that continue to keep you in your current state of pain, which often cause chronic injuries, and all too often *decrease* your performance.

Good training programs should provide multi-step routines that involve both your **neuromuscular** and **cardiovascular** systems — which together develop your power, balance, flexibility, and strength.

The correct program for you involves much more than just a series of sets, repetitions, and tempo with a few rest days thrown in for good measure. Training is a dynamic program that has to change with the responses of *your* unique body, and that meets *your* specific needs.

What's Special About Our Exercises

The exercises in this book have been selected to help you to develop great neuromuscular control, flexibility, power, and strength in your body. These exercises are very effective in preventing and treating soft tissue injuries if they are performed during the early stages of injury or restriction. These exercises are also key to strengthening the weak links in your kinetic chain. These weak links may have been inhibiting not only your activities of daily living, but also your athletic performance.

Remember, if you have a problem or restriction in any area, then you must first resolve that problem before embarking into Performance training, otherwise you increase the risk of re-injuring yourself.

- Use the warm-up exercises to increase circulatory function, activate your nervous system, centre and clear your mind, and prepare your body for the remainder of the exercise routine.

- Use the balance and proprioceptive exercises to develop your neuromuscular control. We cannot over-state the importance of this key factor for both rehabilitation and athletic performance. Increased neuromuscular control equals increased power and increased ability to perform an action with less effort.

- Use the stretching and myofascial exercises to decrease muscle tension, stop the formation of myofascial adhesions, increase flexibility, and reduce the risk of muscle, joint, ligament, and tendon injuries.

- Use the resistance exercises to strengthen your entire musculoskeletal system. These exercises act to strengthen your muscles, ligaments, tendons, connective tissue, and even your bones.

Through our clinical experience, we have found that the patients who follow our rehabilitative exercise recommendations find that their condition resolves much more quickly. So, don't pick and choose only one exercise. Each routine we recommend combines an optimum collection of exercise types that should be carried out together for the best benefit.

Your body is unique and individual - given that each one of us is a unique individual, with specific needs, and unique bodies, you will find that not everyone recovers from an injury at the same rate or within the same time period. Nor will everyone be able to achieve identical levels of athletic performance with the same training program...otherwise we could all be champion athletes.

Some people have a history of shoulder, arm, or hand injuries. These old injuries often create abnormal movement patterns that need to be retrained. It is important to keep in mind that each person will progress at his/her own rate, with the progress being dependant upon previous history, current health status, the amount rest that person is getting, and levels of stress the individual is currently experiencing.

The main point is, that with our exercise protocols, you can achieve great results if you *closely monitor your body's responses*, and then *fine-tune* the exercise routines accordingly.

Listen to your body - if it tells you to rest, then rest. If your body says you have not yet recovered from your injury, then give it the time it needs. Don't just jump to the next level of training if your body says "*Not Just Yet!*" On the other hand, if your body is sending you the message that it can handle the new demands, then go for it. Just remember that your body may change its mind, so listen to the feedback it is giving you!

Keep your kinetic relationships in mind - remember, the focus of these books is to develop and strengthen not just your individual muscles, but also the inter-relationships between your various soft tissue structures.

For maximum effectiveness, you need to develop an awareness of these kinetic relationships as you perform these exercises. Your conscious awareness of the structural inter-relationships (as you exercise) will have a huge influence upon the effectiveness of these routines.

With good neuromuscular control, your muscles fibres will fire in the correct sequence, allowing power to be transferred smoothly from your core, to your shoulders, down through your arms, and into your hands. Without good neuromuscular control, you will find that you are continually wasting energy, creating new injuries, or perpetuating a chronic problem.

Take the time to focus and build that body-mind awareness...and thereby improve your neuromuscular control. Remember... *Neuromuscular Control* is the key factor that determines success or failure in your exercise routines.

Progressing Through Our Program

All our *Release Your Kinetic Chain* exercise programs provide a graduated method for rehabilitating and improving the soft tissues (muscles, nerves, tendons, etc.) in your hand, arm, shoulder, and sometimes the core. Typically, you will work through the following three or four levels:

- ❏ Beginners Routine for 3 to 4 weeks.
- ❏ Intermediate Routine for 4 to 6 weeks.
- ❏ Advanced Routine for 6 to 8 weeks.
- ❏ Performance Development Routines for 4 to 6 weeks.

Before starting with our exercise routines, it is important for you to take the time to determine your current status or stage of training. The answers to the following questions will help you to determine your current level of training and determine which routines are appropriate for you to use. Ask yourself:

- ❏ When did you last exercise on a regular basis?
- ❏ Is this your first time using exercise routines?
- ❏ How long have you been doing your current routine?
- ❏ Are you trying to rehabilitate an injury?
- ❏ Are you preparing for a sports season or athletic event?

Review your answers against the following categories to determine where you should start in our routines. See:

- ❏ *Use the Beginners Routines in this book if: - page 57.*
- ❏ *Use the Intermediate Routines in this book if: - page 58.*
- ❏ *Use the Advanced Routines in this book if: - page 59.*
- ❏ *Use the Performance Routines in this book if: - page 60.*

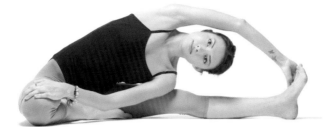

Use the Beginners Routines in this book if:

- ❏ You are recovering from injuries.
- ❏ You have never worked out before.
- ❏ You have limited knowledge about how to get fit.
- ❏ You have taken a long break from exercising and would like to start again.

If you fit this description, then start with our **Beginners Routines**, which emphasize the introduction of:

- ❏ Neuromuscular control.
- ❏ Body awareness.
- ❏ Flexibility.
- ❏ Proprioception.
- ❏ Coordination.

Inactive people often lack the coordination and ability to perform complex motor tasks, largely due to lack of use of their nervous and muscular systems. The *Beginners Routines* emphasize the process of **neuromuscular grooving** where the act of repeatedly performing a specific motion helps your body to learn how to execute that motion well and without conscious attention to that action. These *Beginners Routines* help you to recruit more of your nervous system as you perform each task.

The *Beginners Routines* lay the foundation for coordinating the inter-relationships between your nervous, muscular, and skeletal systems with the goal of helping you to effectively perform any required action.

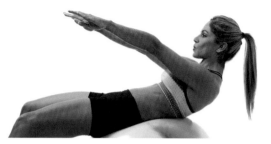

Use the Intermediate Routines in this book if:

❏ You have been exercising three to five times a week.

❏ You have achieved a baseline level of endurance.

❏ You can easily perform the *Beginners Routines* in this book without pain or effort and feel that you are now ready to progress to the *Intermediate Routines.*

❏ Your previous soft-tissue or joint injuries have fully resolved.

If you fit this description, then you are ready to use the Intermediate level of our exercise routines to further develop:

❏ Neuromuscular control.

❏ Coordination.

❏ Flexibility.

❏ Balance and Proprioception.

❏ Endurance.

The recruitment and optimization of your motor systems remains a fundamental component of these routines. This is also when you begin to increase, add, and vary various elements such as weights, sets, repetitions, and levels of difficulty into your routines.

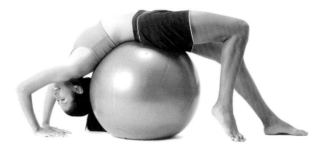

Use the Advanced Routines in this book if:

- ❏ You already participate in physical activity on a regular basis (4 to 6 days per week).

- ❏ You are ready to challenge yourself at a higher level.

- ❏ You are ready to increase the level of performance for a specific sport or activity.

- ❏ You are injury-free.

- ❏ You have already progressed through the *Intermediate Routines* in this book without pain or effort.

These advanced routines incorporate the following elements:

- ❏ Higher levels of neuromuscular control.

- ❏ Increased power generation through the core.

- ❏ Increased strength development.

- ❏ Improved stability and balance.

We incorporate core stabilization exercises at all levels of exercise, with increasing emphasis on this aspect as you advance through each level. For further advanced core exercises, refer to our *Release Your Kinetic Chain – Exercises for the Back, Core, and Hip* book, which focuses on developing all aspects of core stability and performance care.

Remember, for maximum benefits and to prevent injury, you must first be able to comfortably perform the exercises in the *Intermediate Routines* before progressing to the *Advanced Routines*.

Use the Performance Routines in this book if:

❏ You want to improve your level of athletic performance.

❏ You have reached a plateau in your sport of choice and you want to surpass that plateau.

❏ You want to increase your power, strength, neuromuscular control, and the way power is transferred from your core to your extremities.

The majority of the exercises in the Performance routines are dynamic, with a focus upon neuromuscular control. Superb neuromuscular control is what separates the best athletes in the world from the rest of us. Mastering this type of control brings power and precision into each action you perform. It enables your body to generate power quickly and efficiently – without injury, and without loss of power during the transfer from the core to the extremities.

Note: This book does *not* focus upon exercises relating to a single or specific sporting activity. Instead, we address universal kinetic chain elements that apply to a broad spectrum of athletic activities. For more focused exercises, refer to our upcoming books – **Release Your Stride** (for runners and walkers) and **Release Your Swing** (for golfers).

How are our routines organized?

Each exercise routine in our book is set up in the following order:

- Neuromuscular training.
- Strengthening exercises.
- Core stabilization exercises.
- Dynamic and static flexibility exercises.
- Myofascial release.

This order stresses, works, and fatigues the biggest muscles first, and then focuses on working the smaller muscles.

Understanding Repetitions and Sets

Almost all our exercise routines require you to perform a number of repetitions and sets of that exercise. So what are sets and reps?

Repetitions (R) - "Reps" or repetitions are the number of times you repeat a particular action. For instance, when you perform a bicep curl 10 times in a row, then you have essentially performed 10 repetitions of that exercise, also shown as 10R.

Sets (S) - These ten repetitions make up one "**set**". After each set you should briefly rest (20 to 30 seconds) before starting the next set of repetitions. In our books we will always tell you how many repetitions and sets you should do for each exercise. This information appears on the side of each exercise page as follows:

Timed Exercises   **Regular Exercises**

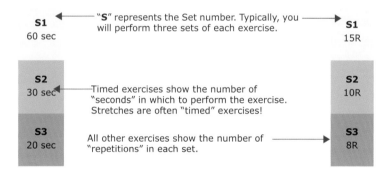

The above graphic appears on the outside edge of each exercise page, and indicates how many **repetitions** you should perform for each **set**. The **S** indicates the number of **sets** and the **R** indicates the number of **repetitions**. If the exercise is timed, there will be a time period stated within the box, as indicated in the example on the left.

Typically, you start by performing one set of an exercise, and increase the number of sets as you progress. Keep the following points in mind as you perform each exercise:

- *How long should I rest between sets? ....see page 62.*
- *Applying the Inverted Pyramid Structure to your sets ....see page 62.*
- *Setting your Exercise Tempo ....see page 63.*

How long should I rest between sets?

We are often asked how long the rest period should be between each set of exercises. Use the following guide to determine your rest period between sets:

Determining Your Rest Period

Training Level	Rest Period
Beginner Routines	1/2 to 1 minute
Intermediate Routines	1 to 2 minutes
Advanced Routines	2 minutes

Applying the Inverted Pyramid Structure to your sets

With the inverted pyramid structure, select a weight that allows you to comfortably perform the total number of repetitions in the first set. For example, if the first set of an exercise requires you to perform 12 repetitions, then you should select a weight that lets you do this comfortably. For example an inverted pyramid training for a bicep curl may look like the following:

S1 – 12 R

- Begin by doing 12 repetitions of a bicep curl in the first set.

S2 – 10 R

- Follow with 10 repetitions in the second set.

S3 – 8 R

- End with 8 repetitions in the third set.

The Beginners Routines focus more on developing your ability to actually perform an action (*motor grooving*) than with the amount of weight you are lifting. Once you progress to the Intermediate/Advanced routines, weight and tension become a more important factor. At this level, you should aim to increase your weight or tension (tubing exercises) by about 10% each week.

Your body tends to adapt and plateau quickly if you perform the same number of exercises, at the same weight/tension every week. When this occurs, you will not increase in power or strength. Due to this, it is essential to increase the weight/resistance of an exercise on a weekly basis.

By applying the inverted pyramid structure (where the number of repetitions decrease with each subsequent set) you also decrease the chances of injury. The intent of our exercise routines is to increase your power and strength by increasing the load placed on your muscles – not to bring your muscle tissue to the point of failure!

Setting your Exercise Tempo

Setting a good tempo for your exercise routines is very important. People have a natural tendency to approach unfamiliar activities with the "*just wing it*" mind set.

Often, with physical activity, people use momentum to quickly power their body through the action. This is not a good idea. Moving quickly or jerkily through an exercise will cause you to fail in achieving the results you desire, since excessive momentum can strain or tear your muscles, tendons, and ligaments and increases the likelihood of further injury. We often tell our clients, "*Slow and steady wins the race!*" This is especially true with resistance exercises.

If you are performing an exercise routine for the first time:

- Pace yourself.
- Count slowly in your head as you perform the action.

As a general rule, when you are shortening the muscle, you should perform that action slightly faster, but take a longer period as you lengthen the muscle. We typically set our tempo at a ratio of 2:4, with two counts for contraction, and four counts for lengthening.

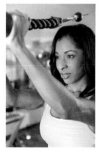

For instance, if you were performing the *Bicep Curl*, you would contract the muscle for a count of two, and then lengthen your arm for a count of four. You will find that by training with a controlled tempo, you will recruit more muscles during the exercise, and each repetition will provide more effective results.

Exercise Accessories and Tools

Although most of our exercises can be performed at home, some of them do require additional accessories or tools. (Most of these exercise accessories/tools can be purchased at www.fitter1.com.) The primary tools that you may need to purchase include:

This equipment	Is used for...
Exercise Handball	Exercise handballs are used to strengthen your fingers, hand, wrist, and arm. The firm grasping action that is required throughout the exercise activates the muscles of the entire upper-extremity kinetic chain. You can obtain different weights and sizes of exercise handballs. Pick one between 3 lb to 5 lb.
Foam Rollers	We use foam rollers in our exercise routines to loosen muscles, release tension, and increase flexibility through the process of Myofascial Release. Foam rollers are a great tool to improve the quality of your tissues since they help to break down fibrous adhesions that form in your muscles after repetitive motions, injury, poor posture, or compensations throughout your kinetic chain.
	By breaking down these adhesions you increase your body's ability to store and release energy. This allows you to perform exactly the same action, but with much less effort. Best of all, foam rollers can be used to release adhesions from your neck, shoulders, arms, back, hip, legs, and even your feet.
	Most foam roller exercises start at the origin of the muscle, and move down across the body of the muscle. When a point of tension is reached, hold that position for a few minutes, using your body's weight to cause the muscle to fully relax.
Swiss Exercise Ball	Swiss Exercise Balls are those giant balls that you see people bouncing around on. They are also known as Fitness Balls or Balance Balls. Exercising with these Fitness Balls increases your balance, core strength, and proprioception. Ensure that the exercise ball is burst-resistant and the correct size for your height. For example, if you are under 5'8", then use a 55 cm exercise ball. If you are taller than 5'8", use a 65 cm exercise ball.

This equipment	Is used for...
Medicine Balls	Weighted medicine balls can help you to improve your hand-eye coordination, and increase strength, coordination, dynamic flexibility, reaction time, and explosive strength. They range in weight from 5 to 50 lb, and are used in our exercise routines for stretching, abdominal exercises, and strengthening.
Exercise Tubing	The stretchy exercise tubing is used for resistance therapy and strength conditioning. The tubing allows you to adjust the tension to suit your current level of strength and tolerance. As you become stronger, you can shorten the tubing to increase the tension. Ensure you move slowly and smoothly, without any sudden jerky motions.
Free Weights	We recommend using free weights (instead of machines) for strengthening exercises. Machines slow your progress and cause injuries by creating abnormal neuro-muscular responses. Machines also give a false sense of strength and power development since they compensate for actions that you would normally be unable to complete with free weights. In contrast, free weights force you to use accessory muscles for balance, and recruit more of your nervous system for better neuro-muscular control. As discussed earlier, the amount of power you are able to generate is directly proportional to the efficiency of your nervous system in controlling muscular system action. Adding extra weight causes your muscles to work harder, burn more calories, and improve muscle power and strength. Some key points: • Select a weight that causes your muscles to tire after three sets. • Allow a day of rest between each session of free-weight exercises. • Move slowly and smoothly without sudden jerky motions.

Frequently Asked Questions (FAQs)

Our patients often ask us many questions when they start our exercise routines. The following are some of the most common questions:

- ❏ *When should I exercise? - page 66*
- ❏ *Can I eat or drink before exercising? - page 67*
- ❏ *What is a Concentric vs. Eccentric Contraction? - page 68*
- ❏ *How often should I exercise? - page 70*
- ❏ *How long do I have to stay at each level of exercise? - page 69*

When should I exercise? - It is best to avoid performing strenuous exercises early in the morning since the likelihood of injury increases after a long period of inactivity (sleep) when your muscles are still stiff and cold. If you want to exercise in the morning, then start with a good warm-up, such as a brisk walk for 10 to 20 minutes before progressing to your routines.

According to several studies, the ideal time to work out is during the late afternoon when your body is at its peak strength.[1]

A workout later in the day is advantageous for the following reasons:

- Decreased likelihood of injury.
- Increased hormones.
- Increased nutrient levels.
- Increased blood flow.
- Decreased metabolism and energy levels.

One of the exercises we do recommend for the early morning is the Cat Stretch which should be performed first thing in the morning, just after getting out of bed. The flexion and extension motion of the spine that occurs during this exercise creates a pumping action which acts to displace fluid collecting in the discs of your vertebrae.[2] This has a positive effect in reducing even chronic back pain.

---

1. Wendy Bumgardner. What's the Best Time of Day to Exercise? March 5, 2008. http://walking.about.com/od/fitness/a/besttimeex.htm
2. Stuart M. McGill, Enhancing Low Back Health through stabilization exercise. University of Waterloo. http://www.ahs.uwaterloo.ca/~mcgill/fitnessleadersguide.pdf

Can I eat or drink before exercising? - Just like your car needs fuel to drive, your body needs a good supply of nutrients to perform at its best! You should eat a light, healthy snack approximately two hours before physical activity (it takes approximately one to two hours to digest a snack). Then eat a healthy meal within one hour after exercising, or have a shake comprised of an isolate whey protein combined with L-Glutamine.

It is important to stay well hydrated while exercising. Take small sips of water frequently during activity. Strenuous activity leads to dehydration and depletion of essential electrolytes and minerals.

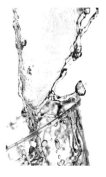

Even a few percentage-points drop in your fluid levels can lead to substantial decreases in performance caused by decreases in oxygen delivery and a build-up of lactic acid by-products. This can lead to symptoms such as dizziness, and nausea.

If you are active and dehydrated, you could get heat stroke – especially if you are outdoors and in a warmer climate. After exercising, drink plenty of water to move toxins away from your active muscle tissue.

In general terms, you should drink approximately 8 to 10 glasses of water each day. Actual amount consumed should increase when you are in high-temperature environments or are performing intense or demanding exercise routines.

Good quality electrolyte-replacement drinks can also aid in rapid recovery. Avoid high-fructose drinks since they have a tendency to spike your sugar levels. Electrolyte-replacement drinks such as Endurox-R4 and Cytomax provide a good balance of electrolytes, carbohydrates, and protein, allowing for increased performance and faster recovery.

For more information about diet and nutrition please refer to the *Kinetic Health Nutritional Program*, available at www.releaseyourbody.com.

What is a Concentric vs. Eccentric Contraction? - The shortening and lengthening of a muscle involve two different types of contractions – concentric and eccentric.

During a typical strengthening exercise, the first part of the action involves a **concentric contraction**, where **both sides of the muscle come together to shorten the tissue.** This is common for lifting actions, such as the bicep curl.

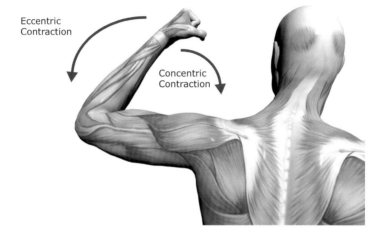

Eccentric Contraction

Concentric Contraction

An **eccentric contraction** occurs when the muscle tissue moves the ends of the muscle **away** from each other, lengthening the muscle. This motion is often responsible for returning the muscle to its starting position.

In strength training, eccentric contractions provide the most effective means for gaining strength and size in the muscle. This is why we recommend, in any individual exercise, that you take more time to perform eccentric contractions, and less time to perform concentric contractions.

How long do I have to stay at each level of exercise? - When you repeat the same exercise routine continually, you will find that your body adapts and that the benefits of that routine diminish. This is known as a *plateau effect*, where your body has adapted to the demands you place and is no longer improving or increasing in strength, even though you continue to exercise.

For example, many of our patients perform physically demanding jobs and inform us that their work is their main form of physical exercise. In such cases, it is important for our patient to recognize that their body has already adapted to the physical demands of the job, and that their work cannot be considered a form of physical exercise.

To avoid this "plateau effect" and to decrease boredom, you should change your exercise routines regularly. This is the main reason we have structured our routines to include increasing levels of difficulty. Typically we recommend that you spend:

- ❑ 3 to 4 weeks in the *Beginners Routines.*
- ❑ 4 to 6 weeks in the *Intermediate Routines.*
- ❑ 6 to 8 weeks in the *Advanced Routines.*
- ❑ 4 to 6 weeks in the *Performance Care Routines.*

Once you reach the Performance Care level, you may want to retain the services of a Personal Trainer or Coach to help you develop additional exercise routines that help you to achieve your fitness goals.

How often should I exercise? - This is a commonly asked question at our clinic. The frequency of exercise often depends on the type of activity. As a general rule of thumb, you should:

■ Perform cardiovascular activity every day for at least 20 to 30 minutes. And yes, Saturday and Sunday are also included in the "daily" prescription. Cardiovascular activity should take place *before* starting any other exercise routine.

■ Perform dynamic range of motion exercises to get your mind and body working together, before beginning any other component of your exercise routine. This activates your neuromuscular system.

■ Perform weight-bearing exercises on alternate days. Give yourself a day of rest in-between to give your body a chance to rest, repair, and recover from the previous day's workout.

■ Perform flexibility and stretching exercises daily. Ideally a total body stretch of 10 to15 minutes should occur at the end of your workout.

When Exercise Isn't Enough!

Are you dealing with a soft-tissue or joint injury that is not resolving from just exercises? Sometimes, your body needs a little more help than what exercise can provide.

In most cases, sprains, strains, muscle spasms, and a wide range of other minor soft-tissue injuries often resolve after just seven to ten days with the right exercises and a little self-therapy. Don't get discouraged if this does not occur for you. It is not that the exercises are ineffective; it may just be that you have built up adhesions or scar tissues between your soft tissues that need to be released before the exercises can take effect.

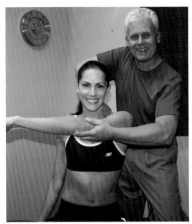

Dr. Abelson using Active Release Techniques to treat a patient.

In such cases, it is advisable to seek professional help in releasing these restrictions.

Look for a good Active Release Techniques, Graston Techniques, or Registered Massage Therapy practitioner in your area, or a proficient deep tissue therapist.

Keep in mind that numerous Chiropractors, Physiotherapists, Osteopaths, and Occupational Therapists may also be trained in these techniques. So ask questions, and find someone who can help you!

Try the exercises first. If you do not achieve the desired result, then seek professional help. Once the restrictions and adhesed tissues have been released with a technique such as Active Release, exercises will once again become a very effective part of the rehabilitative healing process, and can help to ensure the injury does not return. Check with your practitioner, but most specialists will recommend that you continue your exercise program in conjunction with your treatments.

For more information about possible therapies, see the following sections in this book:

- ■ *Active Release Techniques® (ART) - page 222.*
- ■ *Graston Techniques® - page 224.*
- ■ *Manipulation - page 226.*
- ■ *Massage Therapy - page 228.*
- ■ *Physiotherapy / Occupational Therapy - page 230.*
- ■ *Acupuncture and Traditional Chinese Medicine - page 232.*

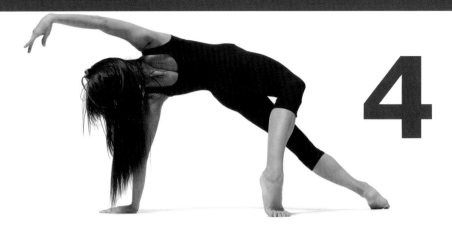

4

What's your Problem...Shoulder?

The inherent instability of the shoulder joint requires us to focus on maintaining a strong, balanced shoulder to prevent injuries and to allow for optimum performance in any sport or other daily activities. To achieve maximum results, this focus must include a kinetic chain approach that involves not only the shoulders, but also your core, hips, and lower extremities.

Your shoulder is the most movable and flexible joint in your body. Most people take for granted the amazing synergy we have between our shoulder actions, arm motions, and elbow functions. This very fine balance between *mobility* and *stability* in the shoulder is what allows us to have such an incredible freedom of motion through this joint.

Essentially, the shoulder is a "ball and socket joint" held in position by a fine balance of muscles, ligaments, tendons, and fascia. This fine balance can easily be disrupted by trauma, repetitive motion (micro trauma), poor posture and many other causes.

Your shoulder is truly an amazing and well functioning structure – that is, until you suffer from an injury that stops you from performing the thousands of tasks that you must do daily. At that point, your shoulder joint becomes the challenge for many a practitioner.

Ask yourself:

- Can you rotate your arm and shoulder through all its normal positions?
- Do you have numbness or altered sensations in your shoulder or down through your arm?

- Have you noticed that one of your shoulder blades "wings out" more than the other one?

- Do you have pain at night that prevents you from sleeping?

- Do you have pain or hear a "clunking" sound when you perform overhead motions?

- Do you have general shoulder joint laxity that is particularly noticeable with certain motions?

- Do you lack the strength in your shoulder to carry out your daily activities?

- Do you sometimes feel as if your shoulder could either pop out or slide out of its socket?

- Have you ever had an injury to your shoulder?

If you answered YES to one or more of the above questions, you may be suffering from an injury to the muscles and tissues of your shoulder. Common shoulder syndromes include:

- Bursitis
- Frozen Shoulder (adhesive capsulitis)
- Impingement Syndromes
- Joint separation
- Rotator Cuff Injury
- Tendonitis
- Thoracic Outlet Syndrome

These injuries can often be effectively treated with proper exercises and, in chronic cases, with treatments such as:

- *Active Release Techniques® (ART) - page 222.*
- *Graston Techniques® - page 224.*
- *Manipulation - page 226.*
- *Massage Therapy - page 228.*
- *Physiotherapy / Occupational Therapy - page 230.*
- *Acupuncture and Traditional Chinese Medicine - page 232.*

By developing good strength in your shoulders, you can:

- Avoid possible surgical intervention.
- Improve your posture.
- Improve sport performance in golf, racquet sports, swimming, throwing sports, and many other activities.

- Prevent and treat chronic shoulder injuries.
- Prevent degenerative arthritic conditions.
- Prevent repetitive strain injuries.

When to Seek Medical Care for Your Shoulder

It is sometimes difficult to determine when you need to seek medical attention for a shoulder injury. The majority of shoulder injuries do not always need immediate medical care and can often be healed with time, exercise, and rest. However, we do recommend that you **seek medical attention** if you suffer from one or more of the following symptoms.

Table 1: Shoulder Symptoms Requiring Medical Advice

Symptoms of Nerve Impingement	These conditions need to be ruled out or addressed by a medical practitioner. Symptoms include: ■ Muscle atrophy or substantial decrease in your muscle strength. ■ Numbness, tingling, or altered sensation in your shoulder, neck, or down your arm. These signs could indicate nerve impingement, and should be examined and treated by a medical professional or a well-trained soft-tissue practitioner.
Symptoms of physical trauma that should be taken seriously	These conditions need to be ruled out or addressed by a medical practitioner before beginning any exercise program: ■ Bleeding. ■ Dislocation of the shoulder. ■ Fractures to the bones of the shoulder. ■ Recent blunt-force trauma. ■ Severe soft tissue damage.

Table 1: Shoulder Symptoms Requiring Medical Advice

Symptoms for Cardiovascular Distress	These symptoms need to be ruled out or addressed by a medical practitioner. Shoulder pain that is accompanied by chest pain could be an indication of a heart attack if: ■ The chest pain is a squeezing, aching, burning, crushing, or sharp sensation. ■ The chest pain occurs under physical exertion, and decreases when resting. ■ Shoulder pain radiates into the left arm or neck. ■ Shoulder and chest pain is linked with shortness of breath. ■ Shoulder and chest pain is accompanied by symptoms such as breaking out in a cold sweat, nausea, or light-headedness.
Symptoms for shoulder infections	Shoulder infections are rare but need to be considered by your medical practitioner before beginning any exercise program. Symptoms include: ■ Redness, swelling, and pain of the tissue with elevated body temperatures above 98.6° F. ■ Swelling of the tissues in the shoulder region that cannot be explained by recent physical trauma. ■ Recent illness that coincides with the occurrence of the shoulder problem.

Note: If you have had shoulder pain for a long period of time, you may have developed some degree of scar tissue (adhesions) in your shoulder. Long-term stress and trauma to the shoulder can result in the formation of adhesive tissue (scar tissue) that prevent free movement. When this occurs, exercise by itself may not be able to restore full function.

You may need to find someone (such as an Active Release Techniques, Graston Techniques, or Certified Massage practitioner) who can eliminate these adhesions. Once these restrictions are gone, the following exercises can help you to regain motor control, increase muscular endurance and flexibility, and strengthen and restore function to your shoulder.

Don't become discouraged if you have a chronic shoulder problem that does not immediately respond to exercise. Sometimes, even a little therapy can make the exercise work as it should. In our clinic, we commonly treat patients with a history of over 10 years of chronic shoulder problems, and find that they have complete resolution of their problems when we combine soft-tissue treatments with the appropriate exercises.

Soothing Your Shoulder Pain

If you currently have pain or inflammation in your shoulder, you may need to first reduce the inflammation with some of the following techniques:

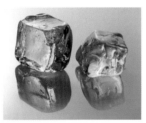

See "Cold Therapy" on page 212.

Apply cold packs - A cold pack or ice can help if you have pain, swelling, or inflammation. Apply a cold pack to your shoulder for about 10 to15 minutes, two to three times a day.

Direct ice massage - This is even more effective than cold packs. Rub ice on the affected area for 7 to 9 minutes. Make sure that you go through all the stage of icing: pain, burning, and then numbness. Your results will only be minimal if you never progress to the numb stage. Stop before you give yourself frostbite.

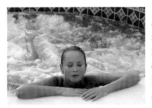

See "Heat Therapy" on page 214.

Apply hot compresses - Heat treatments should be used for chronic conditions to help relax and loosen tissues and to stimulate circulation to the area. Heat can help to increase oxygen levels, transport nutrients in, and remove waste products.

Apply a hot pack (or a cloth soaked in warm water) to the area where you feel the most pain or tenderness. Apply the hot pack for about 10 to15 minutes, two to three times a day.
Note: Do not use hot compresses if there is any indication of inflammation, swelling, heat, or redness.

Exercises for the Shoulder and Upper Arm

The shoulder routines in this book address all the key aspects of proprioception, motor control, flexibility, and strengthening. It is very important that you carefully follow all the instructions provided with each exercise. These exercises give excellent results when they are performed correctly. But when performed incorrectly, even good exercises can cause problems.

We have selected the following exercises to address not only the structure or area that is in pain, but also the kinetic chain elements which directly surround the affected areas of the upper arm and shoulder. The following routines provide suggested exercise sequences that are relatively easy to perform, with a focus on developing movement patterns, muscle warm-up, and activation of your nervous system.

- *Relaxing Your Arm, Elbow, and Shoulder - page 89*
- *Beginners Upper Arm and Shoulder Workout - page 80*
- *Intermediate Upper Arm and Shoulder Workout - page 81*
- *Advanced Upper Arm and Shoulder Workout - page 82*

Speak to your health care practitioner to determine how to further customize these routines for your particular condition.Once you have progressed past these rehabilitative routines, you may want to attempt the exercises in *Performance Care for the Arm to Shoulder - page 101*.

Note: If your condition has existed for a long period of time (chronic), then exercise, alone, may not resolve your condition.
Under such circumstances you should see a soft-tissue specialist to release these restrictions, and then use the exercises in this booklet to prevent the condition from re-occurring. For more details see *Alternative Therapies to Explore - page 221.*

Warm-up for Your Shoulder

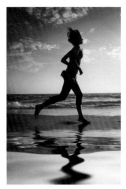

Before starting any of our exercise routines, you need to perform a general cardiovascular warm-up that lasts approximately 10 to15 minutes.

It doesn't matter if this is a brisk walk, a short jog, or riding a bicycle. (See *So What is a Good Warm-up? - page 19.*) The goal is to raise your body's core temperature enough to increase the elasticity of your muscles, tendons, ligaments, and joint structures. This cardiovascular workout will definitely speed your results and help to prevent any possible injuries that result from over-working cold, stiff muscles.

Review —> So What is a Good Warm-up?, page 19

Once you have warmed up, you may want to do one or more of these warm-up massages before starting any neck exercise program to further relax and wake up your neck and shoulder muscles.

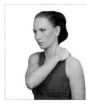

Massage Your Neck and Shoulders, page 110

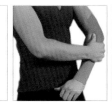

Massaging Trigger Points in Your Arm, page 108

Foam Roller for Your Shoulders, page 114

Beginners Upper Arm and Shoulder Workout

Before beginning these exercises, take a few minutes to relax your hands by applying one or more of the tips in *Relaxing Your Arm, Elbow, and Shoulder - page 89*. Follow up with 20 minutes of a warm-up routine before starting this exercise routine. Remember, to establish healthy motor patterns, you must work within a *pain-free zone* with these rehabilitation exercise routines.

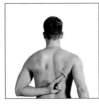
Setting and Activating the Scapula, page 118

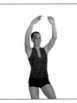
Tai Chi Chuan - Waking the Chi, page 185

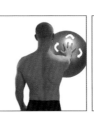
Ball Circles Against the Wall, page 119

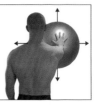
Four Cardinal Points with the Ball, page 120

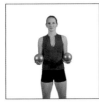
Bilateral Supination and Pronation, page 121

Prone Y on the Ball, page 149

Prone T on the Ball, page 150

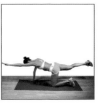
Beginners Four-Point Kneeling, page 155

Beginners Side Bridge – Knee Bent, page 159

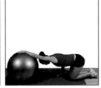
Ball Stretch for the Pectoralis, page 124

Ball Stretch for Your Chest, page 125

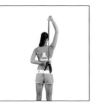
Triceps and Shoulder Stretch, page 127

Intermediate Upper Arm and Shoulder Workout

Do not progress to this level unless you can comfortably perform the exercises at the Beginner's workout. Before beginning these exercises, take a few minutes to relax your arms by applying one or more of the tips shown in *Relaxing Your Arm, Elbow, and Shoulder - page 89.* Follow-up with 20 minutes of a warm-up routine before starting this exercise routine.

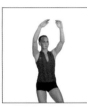

Tai Chi Chuan - Waking the Chi, page 185

Lateral Raise with Tubing, page 145

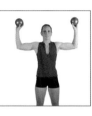

Cuban Shoulder Rotations, page 142

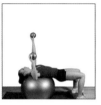

Alternating Dumbbell Bench Press on Ball, page 143

Prone L - Retract Your Scapula, page 151

Front-to-Side Bridge, page 160

Intermediate Push-ups, page 153

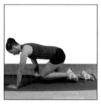

Advanced Four-Point Kneeling, page 156

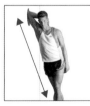

Leaning Into the Wall, page 126

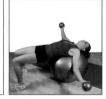

Ball Stretch for the Pectoralis, page 124

Stretch Your Upper Back, page 128

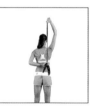

Triceps and Shoulder Stretch, page 127

Advanced Upper Arm and Shoulder Workout

Do not progress to this level unless you have comfortably performed the *Intermediate Upper Arm and Shoulder* routines for at least two to three weeks within a *pain-free* zone! Before beginning these exercises, make sure you have performed your aerobic warm-up (*So What is a Good Warm-up? - page 19*) and have taken a few minutes to relax your arms and shoulders by applying the tips on *page 89*.

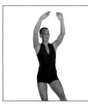

Tai Chi Chuan - Waking the Chi, page 185

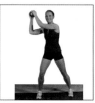

Medicine Ball Wood Chop, page 164

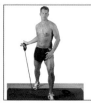

Throw a Javelin, page 163

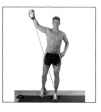

Draw a Sword, page 162

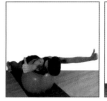

Prone Y on the Ball, page 149

Bench Dips for Your Triceps, page 148

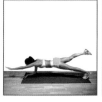

Forward Bridge - Alternating Arm/ Leg, page 158

Front-to-Side Bridge, page 160

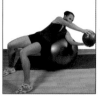

Russian Twist with Medicine Ball, page 161

Prone L - Retract Your Scapula, page 151

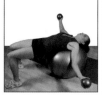

Ball Stretch for the Pectoralis, page 124

Intermediate Push-ups, page 153

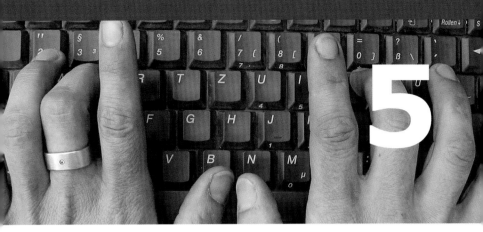

What's your Problem...Arm or Elbow?

The operation of the elbow is directly related to the synergistic actions of the structures of the arm and shoulder. Optimal elbow performance (with a reduced incidence of injury) requires strength, flexibility, and most importantly, full activation of all the musculoskeletal structures involved in shoulder, arm, and elbow actions.

The elbow joint itself is a hinge joint formed by three bones: the humerus, radius, and ulna. Flexion and extension of the elbow joint occurs between the humerus and the ulna. The complex action of pronation and supination (turning of the forearm) occurs between the radius and ulna. To perform these actions, muscles from the shoulder to the wrist must work together. This synergistic activity is a fine balance that can easily be disrupted by trauma, repetitive motion (micro-trauma), poor posture, and many of other causes.

Loss of strength, development of restrictions, and injuries to your arms and shoulders can severely restrict your ability to perform tasks such as working on a computer, holding a baby, driving a car, swinging a golf club, lifting a weight, swimming, shrugging, or even balancing your stride as you walk or run.

The actual structures causing the elbow dysfunction can exist anywhere from your shoulder down to your wrist. In addition, since core stability is directly related to the ability to generate power in your arms, any dysfunction in your core will affect elbow function.

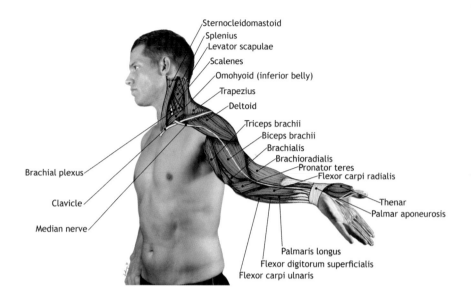

Ask yourself:

- Do you feel numbness, tingling, or some type of altered sensation in your arm, elbow, or shoulder?

- Do you have decreased or restricted range of motion that affects your ability to bend your elbow or wrist, or move your shoulder?

- Does your arm, elbow, or shoulder become sore after performing normal activities of daily living? Or after sleeping?

- Do you notice an abnormal increase in soreness, tension, or pain in your arm, elbow, or shoulder after playing golfing, playing tennis, swimming, or some other sport?

- When you perform activities involving repetitive actions, do you notice:

  - An increase in shoulder, elbow, or wrist pain?
  - A decrease in strength?
  - An overall decrease in your ability to perform these tasks within just a short period of time?

Common Arm and Elbow Problems

If you answered YES to one or more of the above questions, you may be suffering from a soft-tissue injury to your arm, elbow, or shoulder. Common injuries and problems include:

This injury....	Causes...
Arthritis	Inflammation of the joints, usually characterized by swelling, pain, and restricted motion in that joint.
Bursitis	Inflammation, swelling, and warmth in the Bursa. The Bursa is a flat, fluid-filled sack found between a bone and its tendon or muscle.
Golfers Elbow	A repetitive strain injury resulting in pain and inflammation of the tendons and muscles on the **inside** edge of the elbow. This injury, also known as Medial Epicondylitis, occurs commonly in pitchers, bowlers, carpenters and golfers.
Nerve Entrapment Syndrome	Occurs when nerves become trapped or adhesed to adjacent tissue layers. The ulnar, median, and radial nerves are commonly entrapped anywhere from the shoulder to the wrist.
Over-use Injuries	Also known as repetitive strain or cumulative trauma injuries. These injuries result from an over-use of certain muscles and tissues through certain actions that require repeated motions (computer usage, guitar playing, etc.).
Sprains	Ligament sprain injuries are caused by sudden and extreme stretching or twisting of the ligament, usually around the joints of the fingers, elbows, and shoulder. ■ Grade 1 Sprain: Some damage to the fibres of the ligament. ■ Grade 2 Sprain: Partial tearing of the ligament with abnormal looseness (laxity) of the joint. ■ Grade 3 Sprain: Complete tear of the ligament where gross instability occurs and surgery is often necessary.

This injury....	Causes...
Strains	Damage to muscles and their attaching tendons caused by excessive pressure or stress to those tissues. This can result in bruising and pain. ■ Grade 1 Strain: Some damage to the fibres of the tendon. ■ Grade 2 Strain: Partial tearing of the tendon with abnormal looseness (laxity) of the joint. ■ Grade 3 Strain: Complete tear of the tendon where gross instability occurs and surgery is often necessary.
Tendonitis	Tendonitis is the inflammation, irritation, and swelling of a tendon. It can occur as a result of injury, overuse, or with aging as the tendon loses its normal elasticity.
Tennis Elbow	A repetitive strain injury that results in pain, ligament tears, and stress on the **outside** of the elbow. This injury, also known as Lateral Epicondylitis, occurs commonly in racquet sports.

Many of these conditions are caused by the development of *fibrous low-quality* muscles which are full of adhesions (scar tissues). These muscles are unable to contract and relax properly, are weak, and produce compressive forces on vascular and neurological structures.

In this state, these tissues are unable to store or release energy efficiently, thus restricting your ability to perform your daily living activities with a minimum of wasted effort. In contrast, *high-quality* tissues are able to move, unrestricted, through their full range of motion, are not easily injured, and are capable of long periods of work with a high level of endurance. Your goal is to convert your *low-quality* tissues into *high-quality* tissues! You can do this by combining effective exercise programs with specialized myofascial work, and if required, appropriate soft-tissue therapy.

We realize that tissue quality is not something that most people consider as they work through their injuries. But the ability of your muscles to store and release energy is very dependent upon the quality of your soft tissue (muscles, ligaments, tendons, connective tissue).

Proper exercise routines, implemented early in the injury cycle, can resolve many soft-tissue conditions, and prevent them from escalating. However, if you find that exercise alone is not resolving your condition, then you may require some professional help, such as soft-tissue treatments. (See *Alternative Therapies to Explore - page 221* for more information.)

Getting Help!

Effective soft-tissue treatments are able to break the adhesions between your tissue layers, allowing your exercises to become more effective. The right soft-tissue treatments actually change the quality of your soft tissue and can be a key element in injury resolution, injury prevention, and overall increase in performance.

It is important to ensure that your soft-tissue practitioner treats more than just the symptomatic areas that are in pain. They must also treat all the kinetic chain elements for those structures. Ensure your practitioner selects exercises and treatments that address all the affected structures along that area's kinetic chain.

Kinetic Chain Exercise Routines

This kinetic approach also applies to the exercise routines that you perform to rehabilitate your tissue. You must take into account the kinetic chain relationships of the structures that are injured!

The exercise routines in this book take into account the kinetic chain relationships of your shoulder, arm, and elbow. The

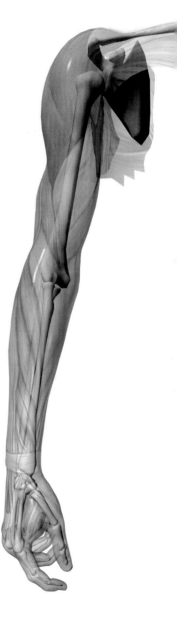

following pages depict some of the specific strengthening and stretching exercises that we recommend at our clinic for the prevention and treatment of arm, elbow, and shoulder injuries.

Exercises for the Elbow and Arm

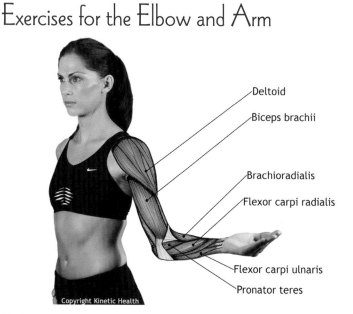

Deltoid
Biceps brachii
Brachioradialis
Flexor carpi radialis
Flexor carpi ulnaris
Pronator teres

Copyright Kinetic Health

We have selected the following exercise routines to ensure that you work not just the structure or area that is in pain, but also the kinetic chain elements which directly (and indirectly) surround that affected area. All routines should be performed in a pain-free rehabilitative state. See *Rehabilitating an Injury - page 1* for more information.

The following routines provide suggested sequences. We recommend that you speak to your health care practitioner to determine if further customization is required for your particular condition.

❏ *Relaxing Your Arm, Elbow, and Shoulder - page 89.*

❏ *Beginners Arm and Elbow Workout - page 90.*

❏ *Intermediate Arm and Elbow Workout - page 91.*

❏ *Advanced Arm and Elbow Workout - page 92.*

Check with your practitioner to determine which of these exercises can best help you resolve your condition.

Note: If your condition has existed for a long period of time, then exercise alone may not resolve your condition. Under such circumstances you should see a soft-tissue specialist (such as practitioners of Active Release Technique) to release these restrictions, and then try out the exercises in this booklet to prevent the condition from re-occurring. For more details see *Alternative Therapies to Explore - page 221.*

Relaxing Your Arm, Elbow, and Shoulder

After a hard day's work, take a few minutes to completely relax your arms, elbows, and shoulders. Massage the muscles of these structures to increase circulatory function, deliver more oxygen to your cells, move additional nutrients to your muscles, displace the by-products of inflammation, and help to reduce overall pain.

Do any combination of these routines, and then follow up with your aerobic warm-up (*So What is a Good Warm-up? - page 19*) before starting the exercise routines.

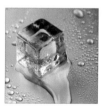

Cold Therapy,
page 212

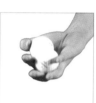

Massaging Trigger Points in Your Arm, page 108

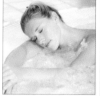

Heat Therapy,
page 214

Epsom Salt Baths,
page 216

Heat or Ice?

Ice Treatment

Use cold or ice treatment for acute injuries. This is ideal for recent injuries (that occurred within the last 72 hours) with indications of inflammation (swelling, heat or redness). See *Cold Therapy on page 212.*

Heat Treatment

Use heat treatments for chronic conditions where you want to relax and loosen tissues, and stimulate circulation to the area (increasing oxygen and nutrients while displacing waste by-products). See *Heat Therapy on page 214.*

Beginners Arm and Elbow Workout

Before beginning these exercises, perform your aerobic warm-up, and make sure you have taken a few minutes to relax your hands by applying one or more of the tips in *Relaxing Your Arm, Elbow, and Shoulder - page 89*. Remember, you must work within a *pain-free zone* when you are doing these rehabilitation exercise routines in order to establish *healthy* motor patterns.

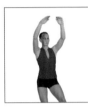

Tai Chi Chuan - Waking the Chi, page 185

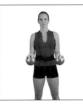

Bilateral Supination and Pronation on page 121

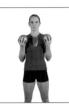

Biceps Curl, page 135

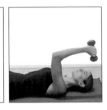

Loading the Triceps, page 137

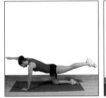

Beginners Four-Point Kneeling, page 155

Release Lateral Epicondyle on Foam Roller, page 129

Release Medial Epicondyle on Foam Roller, page 130

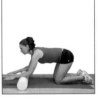

Release Forearm Flexors on Foam Roller, page 131

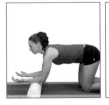

Release Forearm Extensors on Foam Roller, page 132

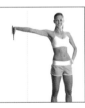

Wall Forearm Extensor Stretch, page 123

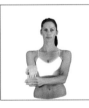

Forearm Flexor Stretch, page 189

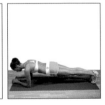

Beginners Front Bridge, page 157

Intermediate Arm and Elbow Workout

The Intermediate routines begin the process of actively engaging your core! Do not progress to this level unless you have comfortably performed the *Beginners Arm and Elbow* routine for at least one to two weeks within a *pain-free* zone! Perform your aerobic warm-up and take a few minutes to relax your hands with *Relaxing Your Arm, Elbow, and Shoulder - page 89.*

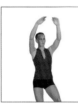

Tai Chi Chuan - Waking the Chi, page 185

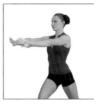

Tai Chi Chuan - Withdraw & Push, page 186

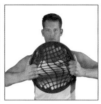

Two Hand Grip Strength, page 197

Handball - Push and Pull, page 138

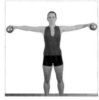

Standing Lateral Raise, page 146

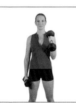

Alternating Hammer Curl, page 136

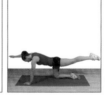

Advanced Four-Point Kneeling, page 156

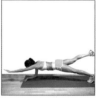

Forward Bridge - Alternating Arm/Leg, page 158

Beginners Side Bridge – Knee Bent, page 159

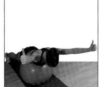

Prone Y on the Ball, page 149

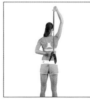

Triceps and Shoulder Stretch, page 127

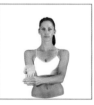

Forearm Flexor Stretch, page 189

Advanced Arm and Elbow Workout

Do not progress to this level unless you have comfortably performed the *Intermediate Arm and Elbow* routines for at least two to three weeks within a *pain-free* zone! The Advanced routines actively engage your core! Before beginning these exercises, perform your aerobic warm-up (*So What is a Good Warm-up? - page 19*) and relax your hands by applying one or more of the tips in *Relaxing Your Arm, Elbow, and Shoulder - page 89*.

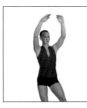

Tai Chi Chuan - Waking the Chi, page 185

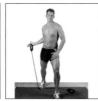

Throw a Javelin, page 163

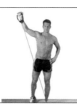

Draw a Sword, page 162

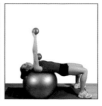

Alternating Dumbbell Bench Press on Ball, page 143

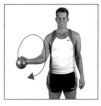

Handball – Elbow Rotation, page 140

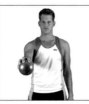

Handball – Make a V, page 139

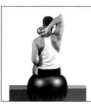

Loading the Triceps with a Handball, page 141

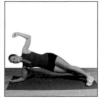

Front-to-Side Bridge, page 160

Forward Bridge - Alternating Arm/ Leg, page 158

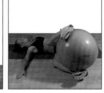

Side-to-Side Swiss Ball Hip Stretch, page 178

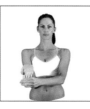

Forearm Flexor Stretch, page 189

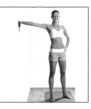

Wall Forearm Extensor Stretch, page 123

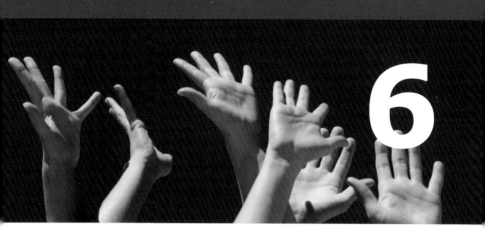

What's your Problem...Hand or Wrist?

Our hands are amazingly complex structures comprised of an efficient system of joints, muscles, tendons, ligaments, nerves, arteries and veins working synergistically!

After all, without our sensitive fingers and our amazing opposable thumbs (the only digit on the human hand which is able to turn back against the other digits), we wouldn't have evolved to our present cultural and scientific levels.

Unfortunately, these wonderful hands and wrists of ours are easily injured. And these injuries can bring an abrupt halt to daily activities such as threading a needle, typing on a keyboard, picking up a child, cutting vegetables, preparing meals, or playing sports.

Ask yourself:

- Do you have swelling or joint inflammation in your fingers, hand, or wrist?
- Do you have difficulty closing or opening your hands?
- Do you have difficulty gripping objects with your hands?
- Do you frequently drop objects?
- Do you have pain, numbness, or a pins–and–needles feeling in your fingers, hand, or wrist?
- Do you get a burning type of sensation in your fingers, hand, or wrist?
- Do you have pain in your hands that is aggravated by use?
- Do your hands have less than normal strength?
- Do you have difficulty performing fine tasks like buttoning your shirt, combing your hair, or holding a cup?

Common Hand and Wrist Injuries

If you answered YES to one or more of the above questions, you may be suffering from some type of soft-tissue injury to the muscles and tissues of your hand or wrist. Many of these injuries can be easily addressed with the proper exercise, and sometimes, therapy!

Table 1: Common hand and wrist injuries and problems include:

This injury....	Causes...
Arthritis	Inflammation of the joints, usually characterized by swelling, pain, and restricted motion in that joint.
Carpal Tunnel Syndrome	Occurs when the median nerve becomes trapped or adhesed to adjacent tissue layers, resulting in pain, numbness, and loss of function. These sensations can occur anywhere along the entire length of the median nerve as it passes from your neck to your wrist – not just at the carpal tunnel.
DeQuervain's Tendonitis	Irritation or inflammation of the wrist tendons at the base of the thumb. The inflammation causes the compartment around the tendon to swell and enlarge, making thumb and wrist movement painful.
Dupuytren's Contracture	Where there is abnormal thickening of the fascia over one or more of the tendons of the hand.
Nerve Entrapment Syndrome	Occurs when nerves become trapped, compressed, or adhesed to adjacent tissue layers. The ulnar, median, and radial nerves are most commonly trapped in the arm and shoulders.
Over-use Injuries	Also known as repetitive strain or cumulative trauma injuries. These injuries result from an over-use of certain muscles and tissues through certain actions that require repeated motions (computer usage, guitar playing, etc.).

Table 1: Common hand and wrist injuries and problems include:

This injury....	Causes...
Sprains	Ligaments are tissues which inter-connect bones at a joint. A sprain is the result of a stretched or torn ligament. ■ Grade 1 Sprain: Some damage to the fibres of the ligament. ■ Grade 2 Sprain: Partial tearing of the ligament with abnormal looseness (laxity) of the joint. ■ Grade 3 Sprain: Complete tear of the ligament where gross instability occurs and surgery is often necessary.
Strains	Tendons are tissues which connect muscle to bone. A strain is a stretched or torn muscle or tendon. ■ Grade 1 Strain: Some damage to the fibres of the tendon. ■ Grade 2 Strain: Partial tearing of the tendon with abnormal looseness (laxity) of the joint. ■ Grade 3 Strain: Complete tear of the tendon where gross instability occurs and surgery is often necessary.
Tendonitis	Tendonitis is the inflammation, irritation, or swelling of a tendon. It can occur as a result of injury, overuse, or with aging as the tendon loses its normal elasticity.
Trigger Finger	When the fingers or thumb lock into a bent position, caused by thickening of the tendon that opens and closes the finger.

Fortunately for you, the majority of these hand and wrist injuries can be easily treated with proper exercise programs that focus on key aspects of rehabilitation and address the main components of your hand's kinetic chain.

Note: If your condition has existed for a long period of time (chronic), then exercise alone may not resolve your condition. Under such circumstances you should first seek out a soft-tissue specialist (such as an Active Release Practitioner) to release these restrictions, and then use the exercises in this book to prevent the condition from re-occurring. For more information, review the section *Alternative Therapies to Explore - page 221*.

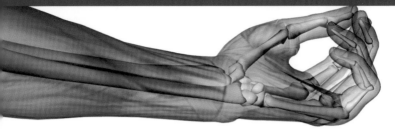

Exercises for the Hand and Wrist

We have selected the following exercise routines to address not only the structure or areas that are painful, but also the related kinetic chain elements which directly (or indirectly) affect the function of your hand, wrist, arm and shoulder.

Rather than focusing upon working on limited areas or single groups of muscles, it is important to plan your training to include the actual execution of the required body motion. By adopting this "action-oriented" training perspective, you will find that it is much easier to improve *all* the affected areas of the kinetic chain. This is an approach which is often missed by many exercise routines.

Keep in mind that your body moves as a synergistic group of links – not as separate components. Thus, an action which initially appears to be an isolated hand motion may actually be initiated by your core (the central support for all upper extremity movements). So if you find some of our exercises do not seem to directly involve your hands and wrist, remember that our goal is to work and improve the **complete kinetic chain** of your hands and wrist, not just the individual structures.

The exercise routines in this book provide *suggested* sequences. However, individuals respond differently to the same exercise routines, and you may find that you have to adapt the sequences and repetitions to suit *your* body's unique needs.

Optimally, you should perform these routines for at least five days of the week to get maximum benefit. Exercising for just three days a week may not achieve the results you want. The following pages depict some of the specific exercises that we recommend at our clinic for the prevention or resolution of soft-tissue injuries of the hand and wrist.

If you are seeing a practitioner, check with him or her to determine which of these exercises can best help you resolve your condition. The following is a suggested sequence.

- *Relaxing Your Hand - page 97*
- *So What is a Good Warm-up? - page 19*
- *Beginners Hand and Wrist Workout - page 98*

Relaxing Your Hand

After a hard day's work, take a few minutes to completely relax your fingers and hand. Massaging the muscle of your hands, wrist, and arm can have great benefits since it increases circulatory function, delivers more oxygen to your cells, moves nutrients to muscles, displaces by-products of inflammation, and helps to reduce overall pain. All good things for your hard-working hands!

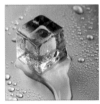

Cold Therapy, page 212

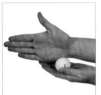

Massaging Trigger Points in Your Hand, page 181

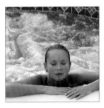

Heat Therapy, page 214

Epsom Salt Baths, page 216

Heat or Ice?

We are often asked, should I use heat or ice to relax my hands? There are benefits to both:

Ice Therapy

Use cold or ice treatment to treat inflammation or acute injuries. This is ideal for recent injuries (that occurred within the last 72 hours) with indications of inflammation (swelling, heat or redness). See *Cold Therapy on page 212.*

Heat Therapy

Use heat treatments for chronic conditions where you want to relax and loosen tissues, and stimulate circulation to the area (increasing oxygen and nutrients, and displacing waste by-products). See *Heat Therapy on page 214.*

Beginners Hand and Wrist Workout

Before beginning these exercises, make sure you have taken a few minutes to relax your hands by applying one or more of the tips in *Relaxing Your Hand - page 97*. Remember, you must exercise within a pain-free zone when you are doing these rehabilitation exercise routines. If you are constantly working through your pain, then you are preventing your body from establishing healthy neuromuscular patterns.

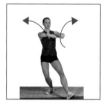

Tai Chi Chuan - Waking the Chi, page 185

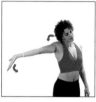

Waiter's Tip – Nerve Flossing, page 192

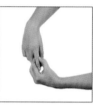

Finger Joint Rotations, page 208

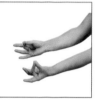

Isometric Finger Touch, page 206

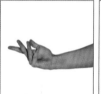

Bharatnatyam Finger Dexterity, page 205

Building Hand Dexterity, page 203

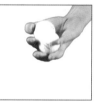

Golf Ball Roll, page 204

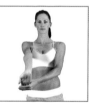

Forearm Flexor Stretch, page 189

Namaste, page 191

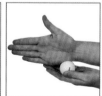

Massaging Trigger Points in Your Hand, page 181

Intermediate Hand and Wrist Workout

Do not progress to this level unless you have comfortably performed the exercises in the Beginners routine for at least one to two weeks within a *pain-free* zone! The Intermediate routines begin the process of actively engaging your core! See *Involving Your Core - page 22*. Before beginning these exercises, make sure you have performed your aerobic warm-up and have taken a few minutes to relax your hands by applying one or more of the tips in *Relaxing Your Hand - page 97*.

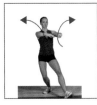

Tai Chi Chuan - Waking the Chi, page 185

Isometric Finger Touch, page 206

One Hand Grip Strength, page 197

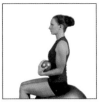

Handball – Wrist Inward Curl, page 199

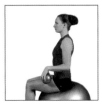

Handball – Wrist Lift (extension), page 200

Lift a Beer, page 201

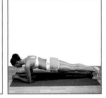

Beginners Front Bridge, page 157

Beginners Four-Point Kneeling, page 155

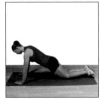

Beginners Push-ups, page 152

Forearm Flexor Stretch, page 189

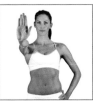

Stop Right There, page 188

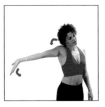

Waiter's Tip – Nerve Flossing, page 192

Advanced Hand and Wrist Workout

Do not progress to this level unless you have comfortably performed the Intermediate routines for at least one to three weeks within a *pain-free* zone! The Advanced routines actively engage your core! See *Involving Your Core - page 22* for more information. Before beginning these exercises, make sure you have performed your aerobic warm-up and have taken a few minutes to relax your hands by applying one or more of the tips in *Relaxing Your Hand - page 97*.

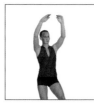

Tai Chi Chuan - Waking the Chi, page 185

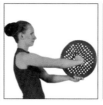

One Hand Grip with a Twist, page 198

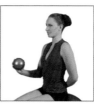

Lift a Beer, page 201

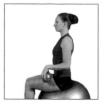

Handball – Wrist Lift (extension), page 200

Handball – Wrist Inward Curl, page 199

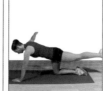

Advanced Four-Point Kneeling, page 156

Front-to-Side Bridge, page 160

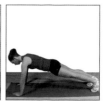

Intermediate Push-ups, page 153

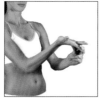

Floss your Median Nerve, page 193

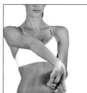

Floss your Radial Nerve, page 194

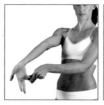

Floss your Ulnar Nerve, page 195

Waiter's Tip – Nerve Flossing, page 192

Performance Care for the Arm to Shoulder

Improving your shoulder's performance is all about building power and strength from your core out to your extremities. It is about establishing strong, flexible links from the bottom of your feet, right up to your shoulders. These athletic training routines achieve results by focusing on the development of endurance, strength, agility, power, speed, and reaction time.

Arm-to-Shoulder performance training is also about increasing your ability to store and release energy. This ability is greatly dependent upon the quality of your soft tissues (muscles, ligaments, tendons, and connective tissue) and your capacity to recruit more of your nervous system. The balance, coordination, and proprioceptive exercises are essential for achieving these goals.

Before you even consider doing these Performance routines, you must first have spent at least three weeks working on the Advanced Shoulder routines. You must also have been injury-free during that period of time.

Performance care is not like rehabilitative care since the demands on your body are much higher, but these routines allow you to achieve greater benefit. With these benefits comes an increased risk of injury – especially if you are not ready for the training. To reduce the possibility of injuries, make sure that you:

- Perform an aerobic warm-up to increase your core temperature.
- Perform all the recommended stretches and myofascial work since they help to build good quality tissue.

- Do not move up to the next level if you find that your muscles are not adapting to the demands you are placing on them. Stay at that level or move down by a level until your body adapts.
- Get some professional myofascial work done if your body is still not adapting, remains continually sore, or is very slow with recovery. Techniques such as *Active Release Techniques® (ART) - page 222* or *Massage Therapy - page 228* can get you back on your workout schedule.

A Workout for Increasing Arm to Shoulder Performance

The Arm to Shoulder performance routines are divided into three main sections (A, B, C), each providing incrementally higher levels of difficulty. Each section prepares you for the next level by increasing the intensity of the routine. Many of these exercises make use of *unbalanced surfaces* or *altered positions* to recruit more of your nervous system for increased power development.

When you perform these exercises, it is extremely important to pay attention to your *eccentric contractions* (the return to your starting position). For example, in a push-up, take three to four counts to return to the starting position of a push-up (instead of just dropping to the ground). You will force your muscles to work much harder, and considerably speed your progress.

It is also essential to work on improving your core stability with any performance level routine. You will never develop true shoulder power and stability if you have a weak core. Development of core strength typically requires involvement of all the elements of your kinetic chain - from your legs and hips, through to your core, and into your arms.

For maximum results, take the time to progress sequentially through all the levels of these performance care routines. The escalating difficulty within each phase helps you to pass each plateau, and move into the next level of performance.

You will be working through the following levels:

- *Phase A - Start with Arm to Shoulder Performance - page 104.*

- *Phase B - Intermediate Arm to Shoulder Performance - page 105.*

- *Phase C - Advanced Arm to Shoulder Performance - page 106.*

Performance routines use the '*super-set*' concept, whereby two or more exercises are performed together, followed by a brief rest. Performing both exercises, back-to-back is known as one *super-set*. As you advance through each phase, you will be performing multiple super-sets to help you increase performance.

Note: The Swiss ball and stabilization exercises are **not** for beginners! Do not perform these exercises if you are suffering from low back pain.

Stretching and Myofascial Exercises

It is essential to incorporate myofascial work into your routines *after* each exercise session. This will speed your progress. prevent injury, and improve your overall ability to store and release energy.

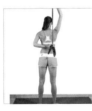

Triceps and Shoulder Stretch, page 147

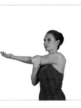

Arm-Across-Body Stretch, page 111

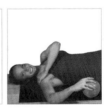

Internal-External Shoulder Stretch, page 113

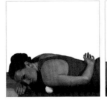

Tennis Ball – Anterior Shoulder Release, page 112

Tennis Ball – Posterior Shoulder Release, page 112

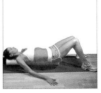

Foam Roller for Your Shoulders, page 114

Phase A - Start with Arm to Shoulder Performance

Start with a 12 to 15 minute aerobic warm-up. Perform the following routines, with a tempo of 2 counts for the concentric contraction, hold for 1 count, and 2 counts for the eccentric contraction.

Super-set 1	Week 1 (1 set)	Week 2 (2 sets)	Week 3 (3 sets)
Russian Twist with Medicine Ball, page 161	10 reps each side	12 reps each side	14 reps each side
Prone Y on the Ball, page 149	10 reps	12 reps	14 reps
REST FOR ONE MINUTE BEFORE NEXT SET or EXERCISE			

Super-set 2	Week 1 (1 set)	Week 2 (2 sets)	Week 3 (3 sets)
Ball Transfer on the Floor, page 169	10 reps	12 reps	14 reps
Prone T on the Ball, page 150	10 reps each side	12 reps each side	14 reps each side
REST FOR ONE MINUTE BEFORE NEXT SET or EXERCISE			

Super-set 3	Week 1 (1 set)	Week 2 (2 sets)	Week 3 (3 sets)
V-Sit Medicine Ball Twist, page 170	10 reps	12 reps	14 reps
Swiss Ball Push-ups, page 172	10 reps	12 reps	14 reps
REST FOR ONE MINUTE BEFORE NEXT SET or EXERCISE			

End this routine with the stretching and myofascial release routines shown in *Stretching and Myofascial Exercises - page 103*.

Phase B - Intermediate Arm to Shoulder Performance

Start with a 12 to 15 minute aerobic warm-up. Perform the following routines, with a tempo of 2 counts for the concentric contraction, hold for 1 count, and 2 counts for the eccentric contraction.

Super-set 1	Week 1 (2 sets)	Week 2 (3 sets)	Week 3 (3 sets)
Advanced Alternating Dumbbell Press on Ball, page 166	10 reps	12 reps	14 reps
Twisting Lunge on Medicine Ball, page 175	6-10 reps	8-12 reps	10-16 reps
REST FOR ONE MINUTE BEFORE NEXT SET or EXERCISE			

Super-set 2	Week 1 (2 sets)	Week 2 (3 sets)	Week 3 (3 sets)
Prone T on the Ball, page 150	Hold for 10 seconds	Hold for 15 seconds	Hold for 20 seconds
Single Leg Lateral Wood Chop, page 167	10 reps	12 reps	14 reps
REST FOR ONE MINUTE BEFORE NEXT SET or EXERCISE			

Super-set 3	Week 1 (2 sets)	Week 2 (3 sets)	Week 3 (3 sets)
V-Sit Medicine Ball Twist, page 170	10 reps	12 reps	14 reps
Single Hand Push-ups on Medicine Ball, page 173	10 reps	12 reps	14 reps
REST FOR ONE MINUTE BEFORE NEXT SET or EXERCISE			

End this routine with the stretching and myofascial release routines shown in *Stretching and Myofascial Exercises - page 103*.

Phase C - Advanced Arm to Shoulder Performance

Start with a 12 to15 minute aerobic warm-up, followed by these routines, with a tempo of 2 counts for the concentric contraction, hold for 1 count, and 3 counts for the eccentric contraction.

Super-set 1	Week 1 (2 sets)	Week 2 (3 sets)	Week 3 (3 sets)
Advanced Four-Point Kneeling, page 156	6-8 reps	8-12 reps	10-16 reps
Lunge with Medicine Ball, page 176	10 reps	12 reps	14 reps
REST FOR ONE MINUTE BEFORE NEXT SET or EXERCISE			

Super-set 2	Week 1 (2 sets)	Week 2 (3 sets)	Week 3 (3 sets)
Standing Lateral Raise ....see page 168	10 reps	12 reps	14 reps
Prone Y on the Ball, page 149	10 reps	12 reps	14 reps
REST FOR ONE MINUTE BEFORE NEXT SET or EXERCISE			

Super-set 3	Week 1 (2 sets)	Week 2 (3 sets)	Week 3 (3 sets)
Kneeling Swiss Ball Rollout, page 171	10 reps	12 reps	14 reps
Push-ups with Unequal Hands, page 174	10 reps	12 reps	14 reps
REST FOR ONE MINUTE BEFORE NEXT SET or EXERCISE			

End this routine with the stretching and myofascial release routines shown in *Stretching and Myofascial Exercises - page 103*.

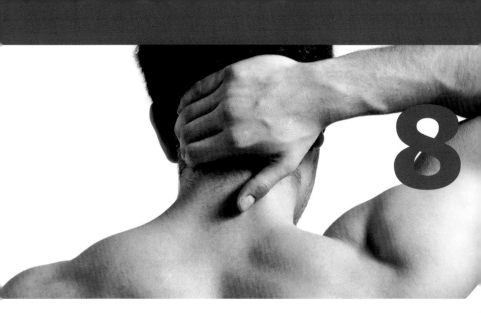

Massage and Myofascial Releases

Relaxing the Shoulder

Myofascial Releases for the Arm and Shoulder

Massaging Trigger Points in Your Arm - Trigger points are tender areas in your muscles. Trigger point massage focuses upon releasing areas that frequently hold stress in the form of "knotted" tissue. Often a trigger point will feel like a small pellet or ropy nodule under the skin.

Trigger points in your hands and arms can cause pain in your outer elbow, back of the forearm, and in your fingers, wrist, and hands. For the purposes of this book, use trigger point therapy on the trigger points of your forearm flexors and extensors.

Tips and Hints for Trigger Point Therapy	How to Perform Trigger Point Therapy on Yourself
• Monitor and record your level of pain during trigger point therapy. Use a scale of 1 to 10. Do not exceed 7. • Ask yourself, "*Would I be willing to do this again tomorrow?*" If not, you are pressing too hard, so back off on the pressure. • Don't be aggressive with your therapy. • Be consistent with your therapy. Perform the trigger point therapy several times a day.	1. Examine your arm and locate the trigger points for the flexors and extensors as shown on the next page. 2. Use a golf ball, and press firmly down upon the belly of the muscle, directly upon the selected trigger point. 3. Maintain pressure for 5 to10 seconds, release for 2 to 3 seconds, and then reapply pressure. Monitor pressure. 4. Repeat this procedure for up to one minute for each trigger point. 5. Once you become more comfortable with the steady-state pressure, try moving the golf ball in small circles to find other trigger points in the immediate area. ■ Repeat the steady-state trigger point therapy at those other trigger points as well. ■ Release the pressure once you no longer feel any radiating responses from the trigger point massage.
After Trigger Point Therapy • Always drink several glasses of water to flush out the toxins that you have released from your cells. • Walk around, or move around to keep your muscles warm, relaxed, and mobile.	6. Follow our post-trigger point recommendations!

Forearm Flexors - Trigger Points

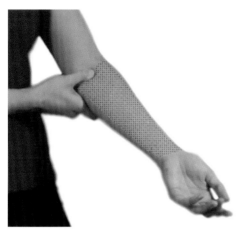

Trigger points in the following muscles show these symptoms:

Flexor carpi radialis radiates pain to the inner part of the wrist near the base of your thumb.

Flexor carpi ulnaris radiates pain to the inner ulnar side of the wrist, and feels like a wrist sprain. It can also compress the ulnar nerve resulting in burning and numbness in the 4th and 5th fingers.

Palmaris Longus causes pain and numbness in the forearm and hand.

Forearm Extensor - Trigger Points

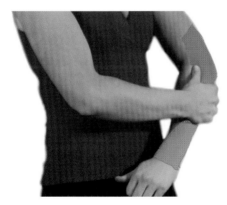

Flexor digitorum causes pain in the forearm, loss of grip strength, and pain along the inner elbow. It is often involved in Golfers Elbow.

Extensor carpi radialis causes symptoms of tennis elbow (lateral epicondylitis). It may also cause pain along the back of the wrist and hand, aching and burning along back of the forearm, and pain along the outer forearm.

Extensor carpi ulnaris radiates pain to the ulnar side of the wrist, and feels like a sprained wrist.

Massage Your Neck and Shoulders - Massage (including self-massage) is the ideal way to relax those tense neck and shoulder muscles that we all have.

Try the following self-massage tips to warm-up and loosen those tight neck areas before beginning any neck exercise routine. Be sure to use some oil or cream if you are massaging directly on bare skin.

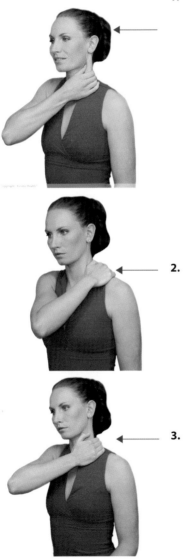

1. **Squeeze and release the sides of your neck:**
   - With the fingers of one hand, reach across to the opposite side of your neck, near the base of your skull.
   - Gently squeeze and release, working along the side of the neck and down the arm to the elbow.
   - Stay to the side of your neck.
   - Glide back to your neck and repeat at least 3 times for each side.
   - **Note**: Do not massage the front of your neck as there are important arteries and veins that you need to stay away from.

2. **Stroke the outer curve of your shoulder:**
   - Wrap your hand around the base of your neck, fingertips touching your spine.
   - Firmly stroke from the back of your shoulders to the front in a smooth continuous motion.
   - Glide back to your neck and repeat at least 3 times for each side.

3. **Massage the muscles around your spine:**
   - Use your fingertips to make small circular motions around either side of your spine.
   - Work from just below your shoulders to the base of your skull.

Arm-Across-Body Stretch - This popular stretch works both the rotator cuff and joint capsules. You should feel the stretch across the back of your shoulder, and in the front of your shoulder and chest.

1. Stand or sit straight. Take your left arm and place it straight across your body.

2. Now take your right hand, grasp the left arm at the elbow, without torquing or twisting your body. You should feel the stretch across your shoulder, and deep within the shoulder joint

3. Hold this position for 20 to 30 seconds.

4. Repeat this exercise three to five times for each side.

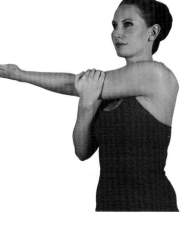

Ball Stretch for the Pectoralis - This exercise targets the chest muscles (pectoralis). Use this stretch to correcting the Anterior Posture that is so prevalent in our culture. It opens your chest and returns your shoulders to a neutral position.

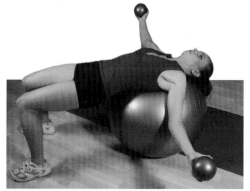

1. Lie back on an exercise ball, with your neck and shoulders resting on the ball, stomach braced, and your thighs parallel to the floor, with a 3 to 5 lb weight in each hand.

2. Extend your arms out so that they drape out over the ball.
   - Relax as you do this exercise, keeping the elbows slightly bent.
   - You should feel the stretch throughout your shoulders and chest.

3. Hold this position for 20 to 60 seconds. Repeat this exercise three to five times.

Tennis Ball – Posterior Shoulder Release - The back of the shoulder often become tense and tight for many people who work at a desk or computer in a stationary position. Use a tennis ball to release tension and adhesions from specific areas along the back of your shoulder.

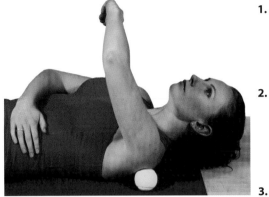

1. Lie on your back, on a carpet or exercise mat, with the tennis ball under the restricted area.

2. Move or rotate your shoulder slightly to cause the tennis ball to penetrate deeper into the tissue.

3.

4. Once you find the point of restriction, keep working the ball at that location for an additional 15 to 30 seconds until the tension subsides.

5. Repeat for each part of your shoulder that feels tight and restricted.

Tennis Ball – Anterior Shoulder Release - Use a tennis ball to release tension and adhesions from specific areas along the front of your shoulder.

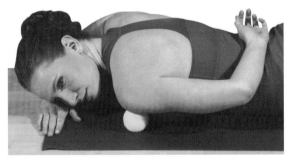

1. Lie face-down on a carpet or exercise mat. Place the tennis ball under the front of your shoulder, and gently push your weight onto it.

2. Move or rotate your body slightly to cause the tennis ball to penetrate deeper into the tissue. Once you find the point of restriction, keep the ball at that location for an additional 15 to 30 seconds until the tension subsides.

3. Repeat for each part of the shoulder that feels tight and restricted.

Internal-External Shoulder Stretch - The rotator cuff, scapulae, and joint capsules of the shoulder often become tight with repeated throwing motions, racquet sports, or tasks that require you to continually reach overhead. This stretch will help to release those structures. You will need a small hand weight to perform this stretch.

A

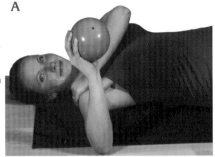

1. Lay on the floor with your shoulder blades touching the floor.
   - ■ Hold the hand weight in your right hand as shown in image A.
   - ■ Use your left hand to press your right shoulder into the floor.

2. Internally rotate your shoulder to bring the right hand towards the floor. See image B.
   Keep your right shoulder pinned to the ground, and do not allow your right hand to touch the floor. Hold this position of maximum stretch for 10 to 20 seconds.

B

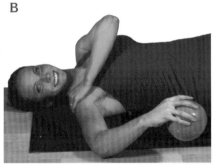

3. Rotate back to the top, and *externally* rotate your shoulder back to bring the ball beside your head.
   Don't worry if your hand does not touch the floor. Hold this position of maximum stretch for 10 to 20 seconds.

C

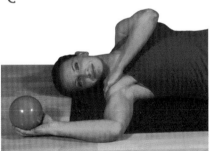

4. Repeat this action, moving between internal and external rotation, 3 to 5 times.

5. Repeat this stretch for the opposite side.

Foam Roller for Your Shoulders - If your shoulder muscles are really tight, you will be amazed at how quickly they relax with the following foam roller exercise. This exercise releases tightness in the posterior and lateral shoulder muscles (serratus anterior, posterior capsule, lateral/rear deltoids), in the lateral chest muscles (latissimus dorsi, teres major), and the upper back muscles (rhomboids, middle trapezius, thoracic spine).

Caution: **Never** use the foam roller along the **front** or **side** of your neck. Several critical arteries and veins (including the carotid artery) pump blood from your heart to your head and back to the heart. Crushing these with a foam roller could result in serious injury.

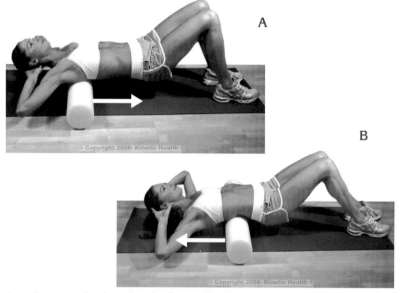

A

B

1. Lie on your back so that the foam roller is across your spine, and placed just under your shoulder.

    ■ Bend your knees and place your feet flat on the ground.
    ■ Brace your core, and lift your hips off the ground so that your body forms a straight line as shown in image **A**.

2. Roll back and forth on the foam roller, from the top of your shoulders to your mid-back as shown in image **B**.
    DO NOT roll onto the sides or front of your neck since you could crush delicate veins and arteries.

3. Perform this action for 45 to 60 seconds. You may feel a little tenderness the next day, but this will quickly pass, and is a good indicator that you have released restrictions in that area.

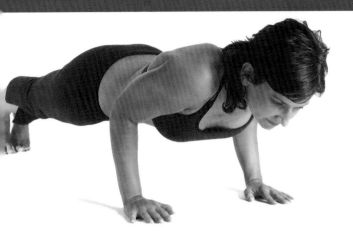

Exercises for the Arm to Shoulder

Body Awareness for Arm, Elbow, and Shoulder

Stretching and Relaxing the Arm, Elbow, and Shoulder

Strengthening Exercises for the Arm

Strengthening Exercises for the Forearm and Elbow

Strengthening Exercises for the Upper Arm and Shoulder

Strengthening Exercises for the Back and Core

Performance Care for the Shoulder

Setting and Activating the Scapula -

Start every upper body exercise with your shoulders in the position shown here. This exercise helps you to build awareness of where the scapula is and learn what its normal positioning should be. You will need this awareness to do the remainder of the exercises in this chapter. Always start with this exercise.

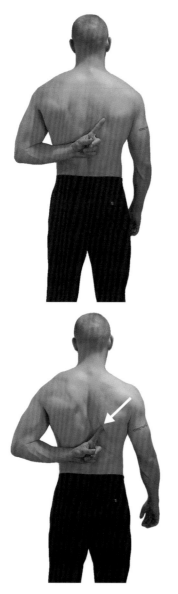

1. Stand straight, with both hands hanging loosely by your sides.

2. Extend the forefinger of your left hand and reach behind your back to lightly touch the medial (bottom inner) edge of your right scapula or shoulder blade. Keep the other arm relaxed.

3. Bring both scapulae downwards and towards the midline of your back to activate the lower trapezius muscles. You should be pushing towards the finger that is touching the scapula.

   - Ensure you do not activate any other muscles.
   - Keep the upper trapezius and latissimus dorsi of your back relaxed.
   - The entire movement should come from the muscles (lower trapezius) pushing the scapula down onto the finger.
   - This is the scapula's *normal* (and desired) position, where the bottom of the scapula has flattened out.
   - Conduct most of the exercises in this chapter with your scapulae in this position.

4. Hold this position for 3 to 5 seconds and then take 3 to 5 seconds to slowly release and return to neutral position. Repeat 3 to 5 times on each side.

Note: Poor scapular positioning will cause the bottom edge of the scapula to protrude outwards.

Ball Circles Against the Wall - This exercise works on proprioception, balance, and coordination of the shoulder and its surrounding muscles as it moves through various ranges of motion.

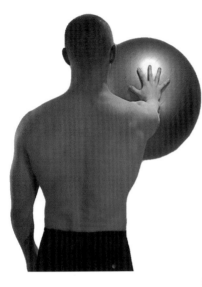

Pick the right ball size for your height:

- 55 cm will be the right size if you are 5 '5" or shorter.

- 65 cm ball if you are between 5'6" and 6'1".

- 75 cm ball if you are 6'2" or taller.

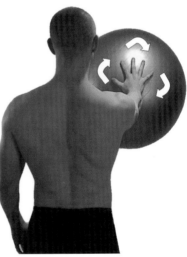

1. Place the ball against the wall – at about face height – and hold it there with one hand.

2. Set your scapulae to its *normal* position, using the method described in *Setting and Activating the Scapula - page 118*.

3. Roll 10 to15 small clockwise circles with the ball against the wall – while keeping the scapulae set. Then repeat in an anti-clockwise direction.
   - ■ Avoid shrugging.
   - ■ Make sure you do *not* activate or use the upper trapezius (from the base of your neck to your upper shoulder).
   - ■ Keep your scapulae activated throughout the exercise.

4. Repeat this exercise two to three times, for both arms.

Four Cardinal Points with the Ball - This exercise works on proprioception, balance, and coordination for your shoulder and its surrounding muscles as it moves through various ranges of motion.

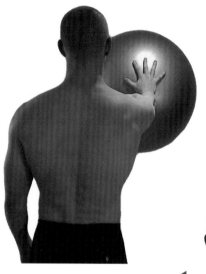

Pick the right ball size for your height:

- 55 cm will be the right size if you are 5 '5" or shorter.
- 65 cm ball if you are between 5'6" and 6'1".
- 75 cm ball if you are 6'2" or taller.

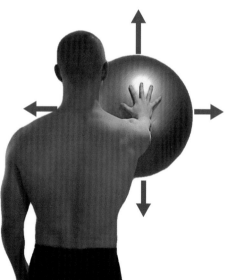

1. Place the ball against the wall – at about face height – and hold it there with one hand.

2. Set your scapulae to its *normal* position, using the method described in *Setting and Activating the Scapula - page 118.*

3. Starting from the centre, move the ball to each of the compass cardinal points, returning to the centre point after touching each compass point.
   - Make sure you do *not* activate or use the upper trapezius.
   - Avoid shrugging your shoulder.

4. Repeat this exercise two to three times, for both arms

Bilateral Supination and Pronation - We constantly use our forearms for motions such as writing, mousing, cooking, hammering, or turning a screwdriver. Sports such as golf, baseball, tennis, and hockey require these motions. To allow us to perform these actions, we need to strengthen the muscles in these areas. This exercise grooves the neuromuscular patterns of the arms and increases circulatory function. For best results you will require soft-weights for this exercise.

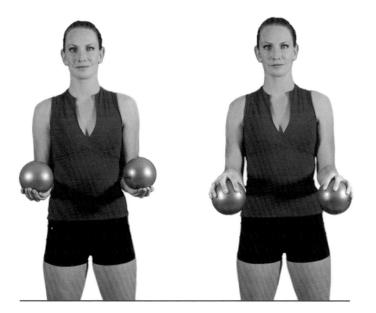

S1
12R

S2
10R

S3
8R

1. Starting position: Stand with your spine in neutral position.
   - Grasp a soft-weight in each hand, with the palms face up.
   - Keep your elbows bent and close to your sides.
   - Brace your core and inhale.
2. Exhale and slowly turn your forearms so the palms are facing down.
   - Keep your elbows by your side throughout the exercise.
   - Hold for 2 seconds.
3. Slowly, for a count of two, return your forearms to the starting position.
4. Repeat this exercise for the recommended number of sets and repetitions.

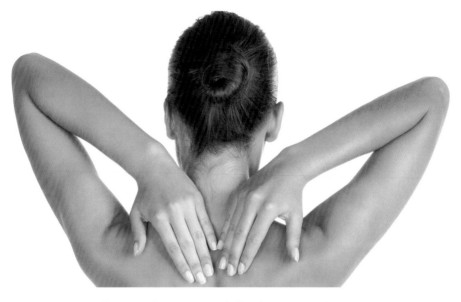

Stretching and Relaxing the Arm, Elbow, and Shoulder

Wall Forearm Extensor Stretch - Your forearm extensor muscles participate whenever you perform a gripping action with your hand (such as holding a tennis racquet) or when you extend your wrist. Muscular fatigue, weakness, over-exertion, or over-use of this muscle can make it difficult to perform daily activities. Use this stretch to relax, and loosen the muscle fibres in your forearm.

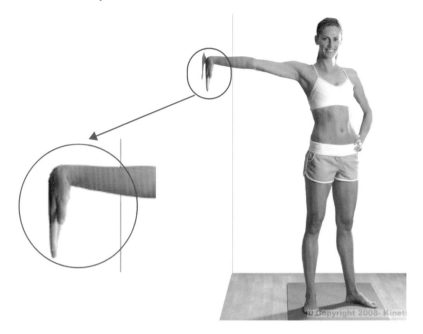

1. Extend your affected hand out to the side, with your arm at shoulder height.

2. Place the back of your extended hand against the wall and press gently until you feel a light stretch across the top of your forearm.
   - Keep your body erect and centered.
   - Keep your arm aligned with your shoulder.
   - Take at least 30 seconds to reach this maximum stretch.

3. Repeat this exercise five times, taking at least 30 seconds for each stretch.

4. Repeat the entire sequence for the other arm.

Note: See *Stop Right There - page 188* for another forearm extensor stretch.

Ball Stretch for the Pectoralis - This exercise targets the chest muscles (pectoralis). This is a great exercise to help reverse Forward Posture Syndrome (FPS). This syndrome describes the shoulders–rolled–forward, neck-tilting posture that you often see with people who work at desk jobs. FSP is responsible for neck pain, headaches, and elbow, wrist, and even hand problems. Use this exercise to bring your shoulders back to a neutral position and help to prevent or eliminate this condition.

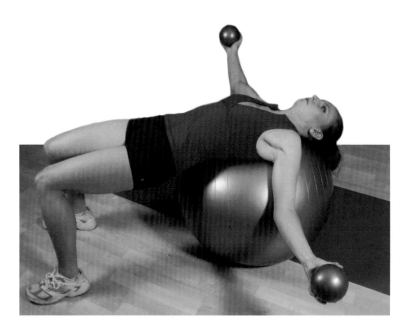

1. Select a 5 to10 lb weight for each hand.

2. Lie back on an exercise ball, with your neck and shoulders resting on the ball, stomach braced, and your thighs parallel to the floor.

3. Extend your arms out to the sides so that they drape out over the ball.
    - Relax and breathe as you do this exercise.
    - You should feel the stretch throughout your shoulders and chest.
    - Hold the stretch for 30 to 60 seconds.

Ball Stretch for Your Chest - This is an excellent stretch for releasing the subscapularis, serratus anterior, latissimus dorsi, pectoralis, and anterior shoulder muscles.

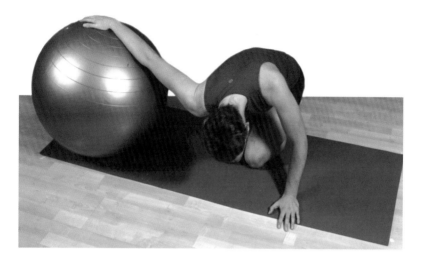

1. Starting position: Kneel on all fours with the exercise ball at your side.
   - Brace your core, and ensure that your back is parallel to the floor.
   - Keep your face looking down to the floor.
   - Place your hand on top of the ball.
   - Keep your other hand on the floor to maintain your balance.

2. Keep your hand on the ball, exhale, and lower your shoulder towards the floor until you feel a good stretch through your chest.

3. Hold this stretch for 15 to 30 seconds before returning to the starting position.

4. Repeat the stretch for the other side of your body.

Note: If you do not feel much of a stretch through your chest, then move the ball (forward or back) until you feel an area of restriction, and then repeat this exercise.

Leaning Into the Wall - This stretches the subscapularis and axillary muscles. The subscapularis muscle is often tight and restricted when you suffer from a shoulder injury. This muscle is used for forehand strokes in tennis and other racquet sports, overhead throws, pitching baseballs, playing volleyball, and in the front crawl when swimming. When this muscle is injured, you may find it difficult to sleep on your side, or be unable to raise your arm overhead.

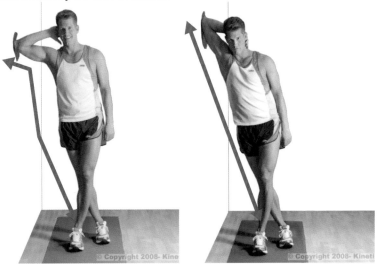

A B

1. Attain your starting posture:
    - Place your feet about two feet from the wall.
    - Cross your left leg over your right as shown in Image **A**.
    - Lean your elbow against the wall.
    - At this point, your body should be relaxed with no tension or strain.

2. **Exhale** as you lean your hips into the wall.
    - Increase the stretch by leaning your upper body **into** the wall.
    - Your body should form a straight line from elbow to ankle as shown in Image **B**.

3. Hold this stretch for 15 to 30 seconds.

4. Now face the opposite direction, cross your left leg over the right, and repeat the exercise for the opposite side.

Attention: Avoid slumping with the head forward when you perform this exercise.

Triceps and Shoulder Stretch - This is an excellent stretching exercise that works a number of muscles including the triceps, subscapularis, serratus anterior, infraspinatus, teres minor, and teres major. You will need a long rubber tubing to do this exercise.

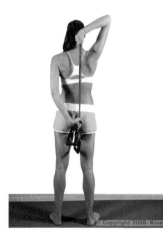

1. Stretch the tubing behind your back, holding both ends firmly.
   - The bottom hand should be positioned at the small of your back. The top hand should be behind the head.
2. Keep the bottom hand relaxed.
3. With the upper hand, slowly pull the tubing upwards as far as you can comfortably stretch.
   - Take at least 15 seconds to reach this maximum stretch.
4. Now relax the *upper hand*.
5. With the lower hand, slowly pull the tubing downwards as far as you can comfortably stretch.
   - Take at least 15 seconds to reach this maximum stretch.
   - Do *not* allow the upper hand to rest at your neck.
6. Repeat this stretch 3 to 5 times for both sides.

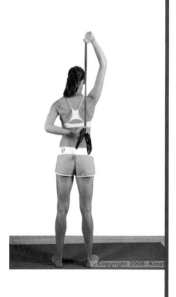

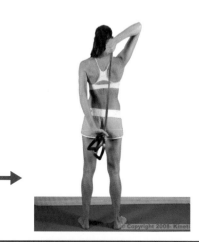

Stretch Your Upper Back - The upper back can often be an awkward area to stretch since it contains many different layers of muscles. This exercise is great for stretching out these layers, including your trapezius, rhomboids, and cervical and upper thoracic paraspinals. You will need a fitness ball for this exercise.

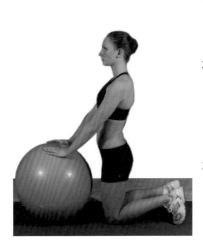

1. Starting Position:
    - Kneel on the floor on all fours.
    - Place both hands on top of the fitness ball.

2. Push the ball out in front of you with both arms.
    - Ensure your torso and head are aligned, face down towards the floor.
    - Inhale.

3. Exhale, drop your head between your shoulders, and:
    - Arch your back.
    - Sit back on your heels.
    - Maintain your hold on the ball.

4. Hold this stretch for 30 to 60 seconds.
    - You should feel the stretch between your scapula, through your arms, and down your spine.

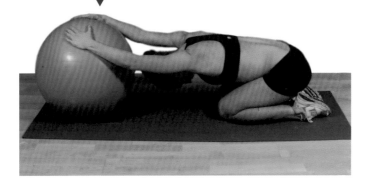

Release Lateral Epicondyle on Foam Roller - To prevent the onset of syndromes like Tennis Elbow, you need to release the muscles in the outer portion of your elbow joint - the lateral epicondyle area. These include the brachioradialis, extensor carpi radialis longus, and extensor carpi radialis brevis. Accompany this exercise with *Release Medial Epicondyle on Foam Roller - page 130* to release the opposing muscles as well. This exercises requires a firm foam roller.

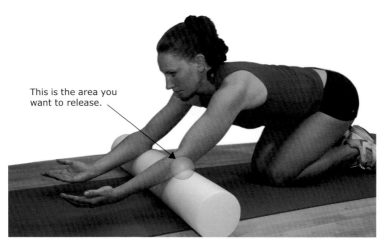

This is the area you want to release.

1. Starting Position:
   - Start in a four-point kneeling stance.
   - Bend your arms, palms facing upward, and place the back of your elbows on the foam roller.
   - Angle your hands inwards, with the thumbs pointing slightly upwards.
2. Start with the roller just above your elbow joint and slowly pull your arms back toward your body.
   - Allow the roller to move across the elbow joint.
   - Once the roller has crossed the joint, stop and roll back to the starting position.
3. Roll back and forth on the roller for 45 to 60 seconds in this area.

Tip: See our YouTube videos for more information. Just search YouTube under *Foam Rollers, Kinetic Health*.

Release Medial Epicondyle on Foam Roller - Many golfers
suffer from Golfers Elbow, caused by tightness in the medial aspect of the elbow. This myofascial release of the medial epicondyle will help you to avoid this syndrome. For best effect, accompany this exercise with the other forearm and elbow foam roller exercises in this chapter.

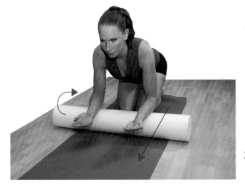

1. Starting Position:
   - Start in a four-point kneeling stance.
   - Bend your arms, palms facing upward, and place the back of your wrists on the foam roller.

This is the area you want to release.

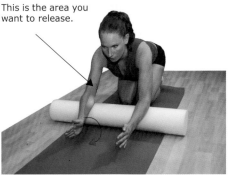

2. Start at the wrist and slowly move your arms in an inward twisting action to bring foam roller to just above your elbow joint.
   - Finish by angling your palms inwards at a 45 degree angle, with the thumbs pointing down as shown in the picture.

3. Roll back to the starting position to complete one repetition.

4. Roll back and forth on the roller for 45 to 60 seconds over this area. If you encounter extremely tight areas, then use the roller on those areas for an additional 15 to 20 seconds until you feel a release.

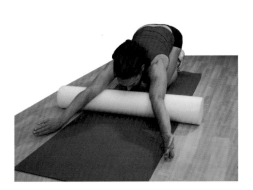

Release Forearm Flexors on Foam Roller - Restrictions in the forearm commonly cause decreased finger strength, decreased grip strength, medial and ulnar nerve entrapment syndromes, and circulatory compression. Myofascial release with a foam roller is an effective way to prevent these syndromes from occurring. Perform the Forearm Flexor Release exercise in conjunction with Forearm Extensor exercise.

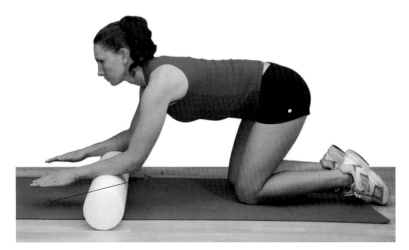

1. Starting Position:
   - Start in a four-point kneeling stance.
   - Place both forearms on the foam roller - palms facing down.
   - Position the foam roller at your wrist.

2. Slowly move your arms forward so that the foam roller rolls towards your elbow.
   - Do not put your full weight on the foam roller.
   - Allow just enough pressure to feel the release of tension along your forearm's flexor muscles.

3. Stop the motion at your elbow and reverse the movement to return the foam roller to your wrist.

4. Continue to do this for 45 to 60 seconds. If you encounter extremely tight areas, then use the roller on those areas for an additional 15 to 20 seconds until you feel a release.

Release Forearm Extensors on Foam Roller - This exercise releases the muscles involved in wrist extension. Restrictions in the forearm extensors commonly occur as a result of throwing injuries, and result in symptoms such as Tennis Elbow, radial nerve entrapment, and pain on supination or pronation of the arm. Myofascial release with a foam roller can be an effective way to prevent these conditions from occurring. For best effect, accompany this exercise with the other forearm and elbow foam roller exercises in this chapter.

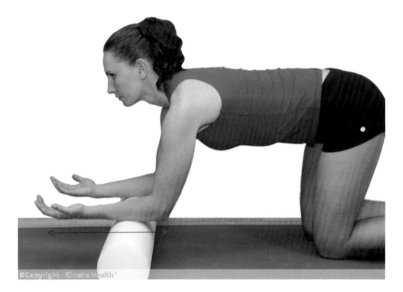

1. Starting Position:
   - Start in a four-point kneeling stance.
   - Place both forearms on the foam roller - palms facing up.
   - Position the foam roller at your wrist.
2. Slowly move your arms forward so that the foam roller approaches your elbow.
   - You can apply more force for your forearm extensors than you would for the forearm flexors.
   - Allow enough pressure to feel the release of tension.
3. Stop the motion at your elbow and reverse the movement to return the foam roller to your wrist.
4. Continue to do this for 45 to 60 seconds. If you encounter extremely tight areas, then use the roller on those areas for an additional 15 to 20 seconds until you feel a release.

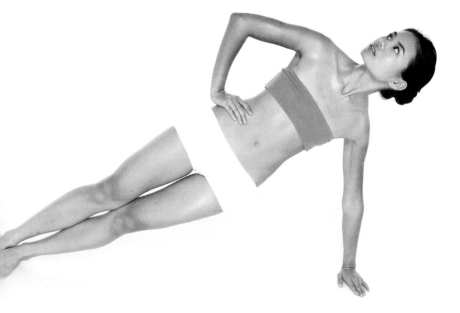

Strengthening the Arm, Elbow, and Shoulder

Strengthening Exercises for the Arm

Strengthening Exercises for the Forearm and Elbow

Strengthening Exercises for the Upper Arm and Shoulder

Biceps Curl - This exercise strengthens your biceps. It focuses upon correct activation and strengthening of these muscles. Use a weight which causes you to *lose* good form after 10 to 12 repetitions. This indicates that you are actually working the muscle to its full capacity.

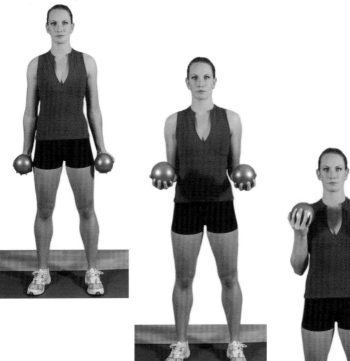

S1	12R
S2	10R
S3	8R

1. Stand straight with your arms by your side in neutral position, feet slightly apart, with a weight in each hand. Keep your chin and chest high, spine in neutral position.

2. Curl the arm upwards as far as you can without moving your elbows from your side.
   - Curl up for a count of 2.
   - You want a quick contraction, and a slow return to starting position.
   - Your palm should always be facing upwards.
   - Avoiding flexing your wrist at the end-range of the exercise.

3. Slowly return to the starting position for a count of three.

4. Perform the recommended number of repetitions and sets, for both arms.

Alternating Hammer Curl - Use this exercise to strengthen the muscles of the elbow's kinetic chain. This exercise activates and uses the muscles of your forearms, biceps, brachioradialis, and brachialis. This is a good exercise if you suffer from elbow and wrist problems.

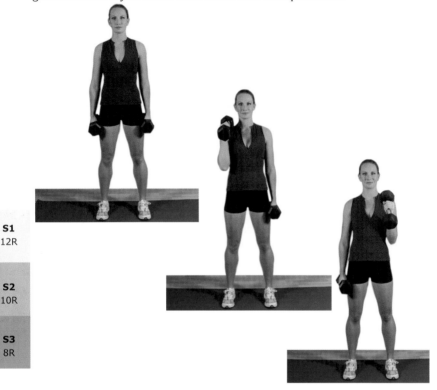

S1
12R

S2
10R

S3
8R

1. Starting position: Stand with your arms by your side, feet slightly apart, and spine in neutral position. Grasp a weight in each hand, keeping your palms facing your body.

2. Curl your right arm up towards your shoulder for a count of two.
   - Squeeze your biceps at the top of the curl.

3. Slowly lower your arm to the starting position for a count of three.
   - Stop just short of a full extension, keeping your elbow slightly bent.

4. Repeat step 2 and 3 for the left arm.

5. Alternate right and left arms for one repetition.

6. Perform the recommended number of repetitions and sets.

Loading the Triceps - This exercise focuses upon strengthening the extensors of the elbow through all its ranges of motion. Use a weight which causes your triceps to tire after 10 to 12 repetitions. This indicates that you are actually working the muscle to its full capacity. Ideally, you should start with a light weight of 5 to 8 pounds, and build up from there.

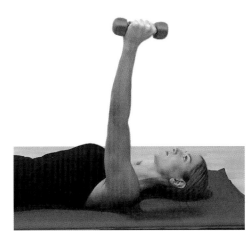

1. Lie down on your back with your knees bent.

2. Hold the weight in your hand and raise your arm so it is perpendicular to the ceiling, and your palm is facing inwards.

3. Bend your elbow to lower the weight down for a count of two, in an arc that ends by touching your shoulder.

4. Bring the weight back up to its original perpendicular position - for a count of four.

   - You want a quick contraction, and a slow return to the starting position.

S1
14R

S2
12R

S3
10R

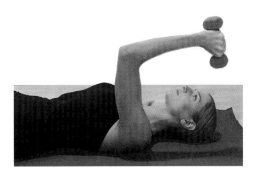

5. Perform the recommended number of repetitions and sets for both arms.

   - Your triceps should fatigue within this repetition range if you are using the correct weight.
   - Perform exactly the same number of repetitions for both arms.

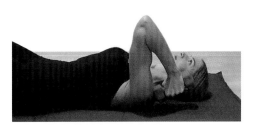

Handball - Push and Pull -
This deceptively simple exercise works the entire kinetic chain from your wrist to your shoulder, and will definitely be felt the next day. This exercise builds strength in pectoralis, anterior deltoid and wrist extensor muscles. This exercise can be performed with a handweight, but is much more effective with an exercise handball due to the required gripping action. After doing this exercise, gripping a computer mouse will be easy!

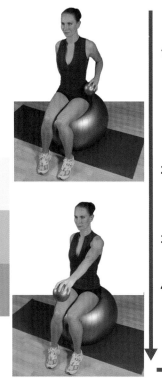

S1
12R

S2
10R

S3
8R

1. Sit on a Swiss Ball (or stand) I with your affected hand grasping an exercise handball.

   ■ Position your elbow close to your side.
   ■ Grasp the handball with your palm facing downwards.

2. Extend your arm forward for a count of two, while maintaining a firm grip on the ball. Return to your starting position for a count of four.

3. Extend your arm out to the side for a count of two, and then return to the starting position for a count of four.

4. Perform the recommended number of repetitions and sets for both arms.

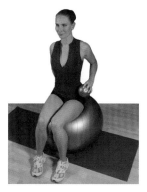
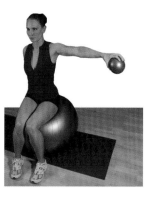

Handball – Make a V - This is another deceptively simple exercise that works the muscles of the kinetic chain from your hands to your shoulder. This exercise can be performed with a hand-weight, but is much more effective with a weighted handball due to the required gripping action.

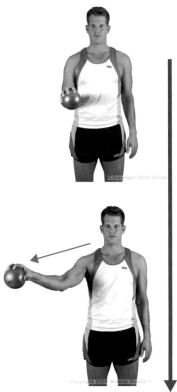

1. Sit or stand comfortably, with your affected hand grasping an exercise handball.

   - Grasp the handball with your palm facing downwards.
   - Position your elbow close to your side, keeping your elbow and wrist aligned.

2. Extend your arm 45 degrees to the RIGHT while maintaining a firm grip on the ball.

3. Slowly return to your starting central position.

4. Extend your arm 45 degrees diagonally to the LEFT while maintaining a firm grip on the ball.

5. Perform the recommended number of repetitions and sets for both arms.

   - Perform the same number of repetitions for both arms.

S1	12R
S2	10R
S3	8R

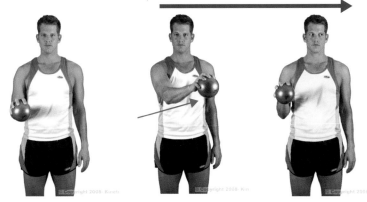

Handball – Elbow Rotation - This is a great kinetic chain exercise for improving range-of-motion, and for strengthening all the muscles around the elbow joint.

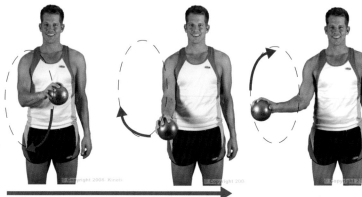

S1
10R

S2
8R

S3
6R

1. Stand comfortably, spine in neutral position and grasp an exercise handball.

   ■ Grasp the handball with your palm facing downwards.
   ■ Position your elbow close to your side, keeping your elbow and wrist aligned.

2. Keeping your elbow locked by your side, perform a circular motion with your hand.

   ■ Maintain a strong firm grip on the exercise handball.
   ■ Maintain proper shoulder position throughout this exercise.

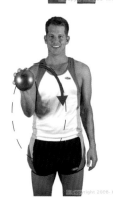

3. Repeat the exercise clockwise as indicated then repeat in the counterclockwise direction for the same number of repetitions.

4. Perform the recommended number of repetitions and sets for both arms.

   ■ Perform exactly the same number of repetitions for both arms.

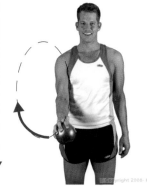

Loading the Triceps with a Handball - The triceps (which means three-headed in Latin) is an extensor muscle that accounts for 60% to 70% of the upper arm's muscle mass. It plays a critical role in upper arm extension, and maintains a balance with the biceps (flexors) when performing pushing, pulling, and lifting actions.

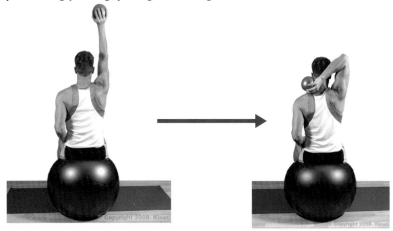

S1
12R

S2
10R

S3
8R

1. Sit comfortably erect on an exercise ball, spine in neutral position, with your feet planted firmly on the ground.

2. Take **two counts** to perform **each** of the following actions:
   - ▪ Slowly raise the exercise handball above your head.
   - ▪ Slowly bend your elbow and touch the opposing shoulder with the ball.
   - ▪ Return to the starting position
   - ▪ Bend your elbow and touch the back of the same shoulder with the ball.

3. Perform the recommended number of repetitions and sets.

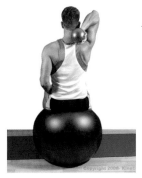

Cuban Shoulder Rotations - This exercise improves the muscles involved in external rotation of your shoulder such as the infraspinatus and teres minor. You need light dumbbells or exercise handballs.

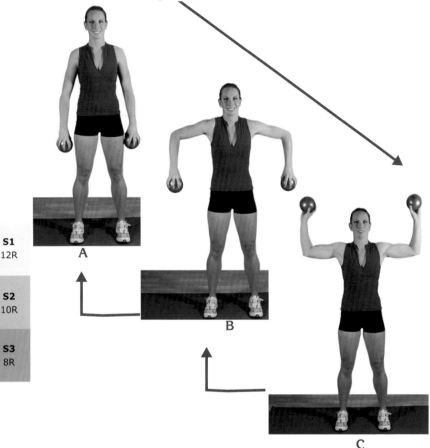

S1
12R

S2
10R

S3
8R

A

B

C

1. With a handball in each hand, stand upright with your core braced.

2. Raise your upper arms to the position shown in Image B.

3. Exhale, and pivot your shoulders and arms upwards to the "*I give up*" position shown in Image C.

4. Pivot your arms downwards to return to Figure B, and then drop your arms down to your side to return to the starting position in Image A.

5. Perform the recommended number of repetitions and sets. Increase the intensity of the exercise by increasing the weights in your hands.

Alternating Dumbbell Bench Press on Ball - This is an excellent exercise for your chest, anterior shoulder, and triceps. The independent hand actions make it more effective than a standard barbell press since the independent arm actions cause you to work harder to stabilize your shoulders. Start with a weight that you can comfortably lift at least ten times. Remember, bench presses are harder than a simple lift of a weight, so choose a slightly lighter weight to start.

A

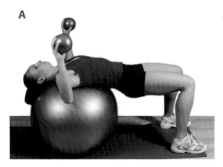

B

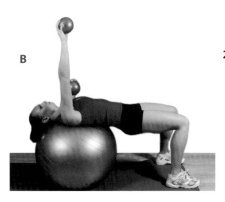

C

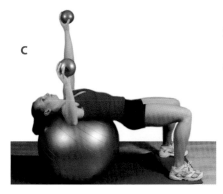

1. Starting Position: Sit on the exercise ball with the weights in your hands.

   - Slowly walk out into a "bridge" position where your back and shoulders are resting on the ball as shown in figure A, forming a straight plank to your knees.
   - Brace your core and lower the weights to the starting position shown in image A.

2. With alternating arms, push the weight upward in a triangular pattern.

   - At the top-most position, your elbow should remain slightly bent, with the weight aligned over your chin.
   - Raise your arm for two counts, and then slowly lower your arm for three counts.

3. Return to the starting position, and repeat for the other arm.

4. Perform the recommended number of repetitions and sets.

S1
12R

S2
10R

S3
8R

Lateral Raise on a Ball

Lateral Raise on a Ball - This is a very effective beginners exercise for strengthening the medial deltoids, posterior deltoids, and the upper trapezius, as well as for developing your proprioceptive balance.

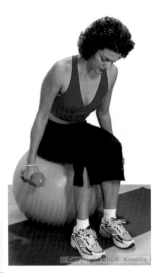

1. Hold the dumbbells in your hands and seat yourself on the exercise ball.
    - Lean forward slightly but keep your back, neck, and head aligned.
    - Plant your feet firmly on the ground.
    - Take a deep breath.

2. Exhale, and raise both arms straight out to the sides, up to shoulder height.
    - Hold the raised position for two counts.
    - Maintain the slight forward-leaning position.
    - Keep your elbows slightly bent.

3. Slowly lower the weights to the starting position for a count of three, inhaling as you do so.

4. Perform the recommended number of repetitions and sets.

S1
10R

S2
8R

S3
6R

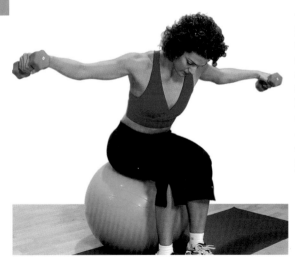

Note: Advanced users can try this exercise with only one leg planted on the ground.
But you must be confident of your ability to balance on the ball with just one leg!

Lateral Raise with Tubing - This **intermediate** level exercise strengthens the serratus anterior and latissimus dorsi muscles. The serratus anterior muscle is responsible for the protraction of the scapula. The latissimus dorsi is a large back muscle, and helps to pull your upper arms down and in front of your body, as well as allowing you to rotate your upper arm inward.

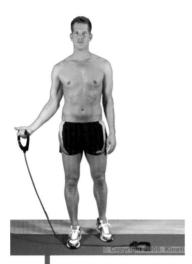

1. Stand on the tubing so that it is secure under your foot, and cannot snap out.

2. Hold the handle with your right hand, palm facing upwards, thumb up.

3. Exhale, and lift your arms straight up and out from the side of your body.
   - Keep your elbows partially bent.
   - Beginners: Only raise the tubing to your shoulder height.
   - Advanced: raise the tubing above your head.

4. Return to the starting position.

5. Perform the recommended number of repetitions and sets equally for each side.

S1
12R

S2
10R

S3
8R

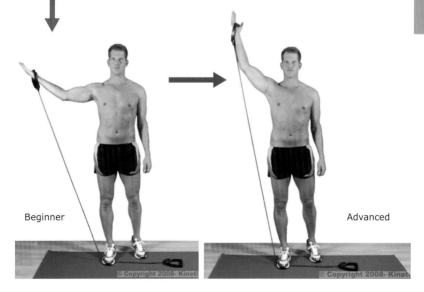

Beginner

Advanced

Standing Lateral Raise

Standing Lateral Raise - This is a very effective **advanced** exercise for strengthening the medial deltoids, posterior deltoids, supraspinatus, and upper trapezius. In the standing position, you activate more of your core muscles and work additional muscle groups.

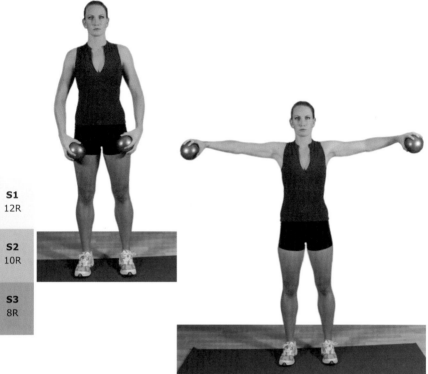

S1
12R

S2
10R

S3
8R

1. Starting Position:
    - Stand with your feet shoulder-width apart, spine in neutral position, with the weights in your hands.
    - Hold the weights with an overhand grip, palms facing downwards.
    - Keep your knees slightly bent.

2. Exhale, and raise both the dumbbells laterally in an arc-like motion until your arms are parallel to the floor.
    - Hold the raised position for a count of three.
    - Keep your elbows slightly bent for the entire motion.

3. Slowly lower the weights to the starting position for a count of four, inhaling as you do so.

4. Perform the recommended number of repetitions and sets.

Handball Rotation - This beginner level exercise strengthens the internal and external rotators of the shoulder. The infraspinatus and teres minor muscles externally rotate the arm, and the subscapularis, latissimus dorsi, and teres major muscles internally rotates the arm. But it is equally important to balance the development of these large muscle groups by strengthening the internal rotators (infraspinatus and teres minor).

Note: Much of the benefit of this exercise is derived from the special soft weight (handball) of about 5 to 8 lb. The firm grip required to hold this ball causes activation of muscle groups from the shoulder all the way to the fingers – more areas than a traditional dumbbell weight – and is also excellent for balance and stabilization training.

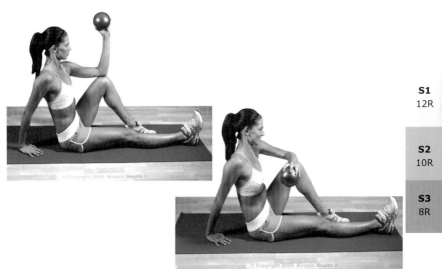

S1
12R

S2
10R

S3
8R

1. Sit on the floor, with one hand on the ground, and the opposite knee bent.

2. Pick up the weight with the other hand and prop this arm up on the raised knee. Your arm should be bent at the elbow to 90 degrees, pointing up to the ceiling.

3. Keep your arm bent to 90 degrees and slowly rotate inward for a count of three until the forearm is parallel to the ground.

4. Slowly rotate back to the starting position without pausing, for a count of four.

5. Perform the recommended number of repetitions and sets equally for both sides in order to balance both sides of your body.

Bench Dips for Your Triceps - Your triceps are often forgotten, in comparison to their much vaunted bicep cousins, but they need to be strengthened in order to counter-balance the power required by the biceps. You will need a secure, non-moving bench for this exercise.

A

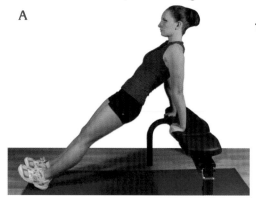

1. Position your hands shoulder-width apart on a secure, unmoving bench. Move your feet away from the bench as far as you can so that you are in the position shown in Image A. Keep your arm slightly bent to prevent them from locking and to reduce stress on your elbow joints.

S1
8R

B

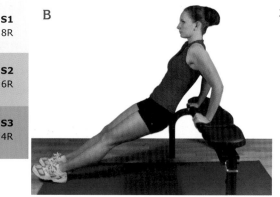

2. Exhale, and slowly lower your body towards the floor. Keep your elbows tucked in; do not allow them to flare out. Your shoulder strength and shoulder joint function will determine how far down you are able to drop. Optimal position is to have your shoulder joint just below your elbow.

S2
6R

S3
4R

C

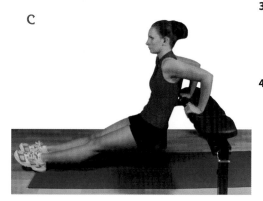

3. Now, press upwards with your hands and triceps to push yourself back to the starting position.

4. Perform the recommended number of repetitions and sets within a pain-free zone.

Prone Y on the Ball - This exercise focuses upon the trapezius, rhomboids, rotator cuff, and paraspinal muscles of your upper back. It also increases neuromuscular performance and acts to stabilize the scapula which performs a critical role in the biomechanics of your shoulder. This is a great exercise for safeguarding against shoulder injuries.

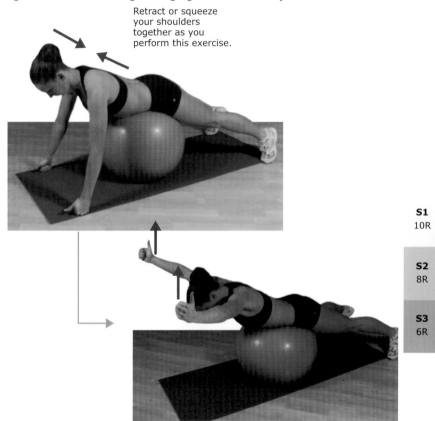

Retract or squeeze your shoulders together as you perform this exercise.

S1
10R

S2
8R

S3
6R

1. Position yourself on an exercise ball, face down, feet and hands anchored to the floor, bracing your body.

2. Extend both arms over your head to form a Y shape. Pull your shoulder blades together and maintain that position throughout the exercise. Brace your core and exhale.

3. Hold the raised pose for a count of two. You should feel the muscles between your shoulder blades working.

4. Slowly lower your arms to the starting position, and relax your shoulder blades.

5. Perform the recommended number of sets and repetitions.

Prone T on the Ball - This exercise focuses upon strengthening the rhomboids, deltoids, trapezius, scapula, and paraspinal muscles of your upper back. After an injury it is essential to strengthen and re-train the scapula since it is a key link in the shoulder and is actively involved in retraction, protraction, and upward and downward rotation, as well as elevation and depression of the shoulder.

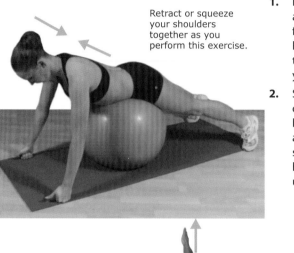

Retract or squeeze your shoulders together as you perform this exercise.

1. Position yourself on an exercise ball, face down, feet and hands anchored to the floor, bracing your body.

2. Stretch both arms out to the sides, keeping them aligned with your shoulder, with your hands in a thumbs-up position

S1
10R

S2
8R

S3
6R

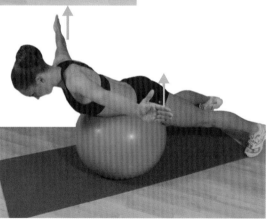

3. Pull your shoulder blades together and maintain that position throughout the exercise. Brace your core and exhale.

4. Hold the raised pose for a count of two. Maintain a slight bend at the elbow.

5. Slowly lower your arms to the starting position, and relax your shoulder blades.

6. Perform the recommended number of sets and repetitions.

Prone L - Retract Your Scapula - This exercise focuses upon strengthening the rhomboids, posterior deltoids, rotator cuff, scapula, and paraspinals of the upper back. The rhomboid muscles are often overworked when carrying heavy loads, and engaging in rowing and racquet sports.

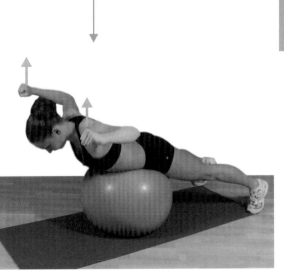

Retract or squeeze your shoulders together as you perform this exercise.

1. Position yourself on an exercise ball, face down, feet and hands anchored to the floor, bracing your body.

2. Raise both arms off the floor, and try and hold the raised pose for a count of two, keeping the arms aligned with your shoulders.

3. Slowly lower your arms to the starting position, and relax your shoulder blades.

4. Perform the recommended number of sets and repetitions.

S1
10R

S2
8R

S3
6R

Beginners Push-ups - Push-ups are a great core exercise that help to improve total body fitness. Push-ups strengthen the chest (pectoralis minor and major), triceps, and the anterior deltoids, while simultaneously stretching the biceps and back muscles. They are also very good for improving core stabilty.

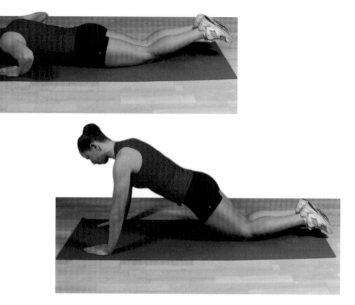

S1
8R

S2
6R

S3
4R

1. Lie face down, palms flat by your shoulder, hands slightly more than shoulder- width apart, and supporting your body weight.

   ■ Bend your knees.
   ■ Brace your core as shown in *Bracing Your Core - page 23.*

2. Exhale, straighten your arms, and push UP off the floor for a count of two.

   ■ Keep your palms fixed at the same position.
   ■ Keep your knees on the ground.
   ■ Do not bend or arch your neck or torso.
   ■ Push up until your arms are straight, but not hyper-extended.

3. Lower yourself for a count of three to return to your starting position.

4. Repeat this exercise for the recommended number of sets and repetitions.

Tip: Once you can comfortably perform 15 to 20 beginners push-ups, you can advance to the Intermediate push-up shown on page 153.

Intermediate Push-ups - This intermediate level push-up increases the lever of resistance to further strengthen the arm, upper body, and shoulder. You should feel its effects in your chest (pectorals), back of your arms (triceps), shoulders (deltoids), and rotator cuff muscles.

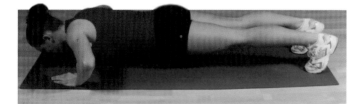

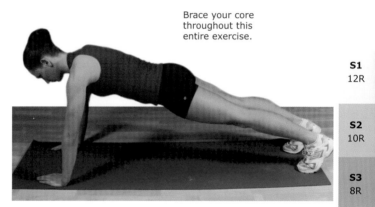

Brace your core throughout this entire exercise.

S1
12R

S2
10R

S3
8R

1. Lie chest down, palms flat by your shoulder, and just a little more than shoulder-width apart. Take a deep breath, and place your toes on the floor in preparation for a plank position.

2. Exhale, straighten your arms, and push up off the floor.
   - Keep your palms fixed at the same position.
   - Do not bend or arch your back.

3. Hold the pushed-up position for a count of two, then lower your chest to the floor for a count of three until your arms are bent to a 90-degree angle.

4. Rest for a count of one, and repeat from Step 2 for the recommended number of repetitions and sets.

Note: Once these become too easy, you can prop your feet up on a stability ball or bench, or raise one leg off the ground to make the push-ups more challenging.

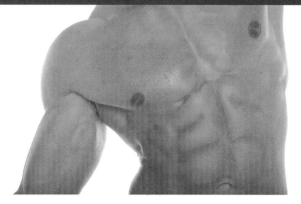

Strengthening the Back and Core

It is essential to work on improving your core stability in order to develop true shoulder power. Core strength is a critical element in both rehabilitation and sports performance.

Development of core strength typically requires involvement of all the elements of your kinetic chain - from your legs and hips, through to your core, and into your arms.

Beginners Four-Point Kneeling - This is not only a great core exercise, but it is also an excellent exercise for grooving your neuromuscular system. Four-point kneeling teaches your body to transfer energy from your lower extremity through your core to the upper extremity. Best of all, it acts to increase the stability and motor control of your whole body!

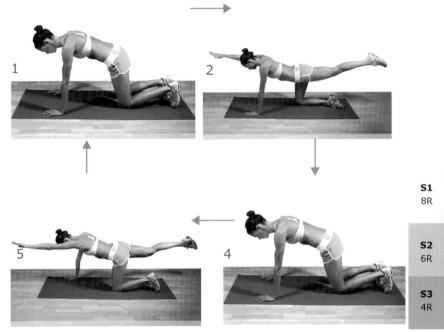

S1
8R

S2
6R

S3
4R

1. Starting position: Kneel on all fours.
   - Keep your hands and knees planted firmly on the ground as you face forward, with the spine in neutral position.
   - Inhale and brace your core.
2. Exhale and slowly straighten the **right arm and left leg**.
   - Your arm and leg should be parallel to the floor.
   - Your arm and leg should be aligned with your torso.
   - Maintain your spine in neutral position
   - Avoid tilting your back and pelvis.
3. Hold this position for 5 to 10 seconds.
4. Slowly lower the arm and leg to the starting position.
5. Repeat the above procedures from Step 1 for the opposite side with the **left arm and right leg**.
6. Repeat the entire sequence for the defined number of sets and repetitions.

Advanced Four-Point Kneeling - This advanced version increases both shoulder and core stability, allowing you to direct more power from your core to your extremities. This exercise improves the strength of the rectus abdominis, gluteals and hamstring muscles.

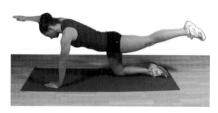

1. Starting position: Kneel on all fours on the floor as in *Beginners Four-Point Kneeling - page 155*.

2. Exhale and slowly straighten the **right arm and left leg**.
   - Your arm and leg should be parallel to the floor and aligned with your torso.
   - Maintain your spine in neutral position.
   - Avoid tilting or twisting your back and pelvis.
   - Hold this position for two seconds.

S1
10R

S2
8R

S3
6R

3. Now curve the extended arm under your body while tucking in the extended knee to touch your curved arm. Don't touch the floor. Hold this position for two seconds.

4. Now flex the right arm out so that it is perpendicular to the body, and extend the left leg. Hold this position for two seconds.

5. Slowly return your arm and leg to the starting position.

6. Repeat the above procedures from Step 1 for the opposite side with the **left arm and right leg**.

7. Repeat the entire sequence for the defined number of sets and repetitions.

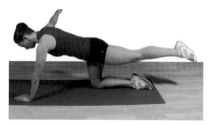

Beginners Front Bridge - The Front Bridge, or Plank, is a classic exercise for stabilizing the shoulder and strengthening the muscles of your core. Ensure that you only do this exercise within your pain-free zone.

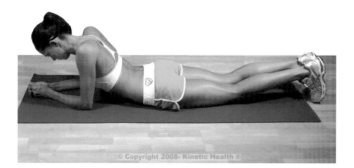

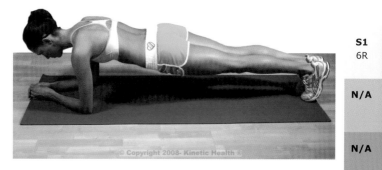

S1
6R

N/A

N/A

1. Lay flat on your stomach with your legs fully extended.
    - ▪ Place your elbows shoulder-width apart, fingers pointing towards your head.
    - ▪ Brace your core and inhale.

2. Lift your body up off the ground so that only your forearms and toes are supporting the weight of your body.
    - ▪ Your body should form a straight line, from your head to your toes.
    - ▪ Do not allow your spine to curve down or up.
    - ▪ Do not sag, and always continue to brace your core.
    - ▪ Keep your shoulders relaxed and do not hunch.
    - ▪ Lengthen your body through your spine as you exhale.

3. Hold the bridge for 10 seconds, then slowly lower yourself back to the ground.

4. Repeat this exercise for the recommended number of repetitions and sets.

Forward Bridge - Alternating Arm/Leg - This advanced forward bridge alternates movements of the hands and legs while in the Plank position. This difficult exercise should not be attempted until you have mastered the Beginners Front Bridge. This is a very good exercise for your core, shoulders, and lower extremities. It also serves to increase neuromuscular control and rotary stability.

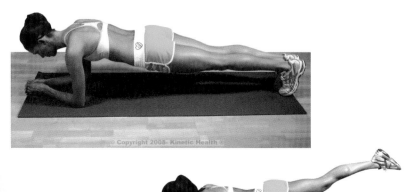

S1
60
sec

S2
50
sec

S3
30
sec

1. Assume the plank position detailed in *Beginners Front Bridge - page 157*. Hold this position for 60 seconds, keeping your core braced and your neck aligned with your spine. Widen your feet if you are having problems balancing.

2. Now raise your **left arm** and **right leg** so that they are aligned with your body. Balance your body weight between your bent elbows and your feet. Keep breathing! Hold this extended position for two seconds.

3. Return to the starting position in Step 1.

4. Now raise the **right arm** and **left leg** and hold this extended position for another two seconds. Return to the starting position to complete this repetition.

5. Repeat the entire sequence for the recommended number of sets and repetitions.

Beginners Side Bridge – Knee Bent - This very effective exercise targets your strengthen the abdominals, paraspinals, and shoulder muscles. It strengthens your core and develops neuromuscular control.

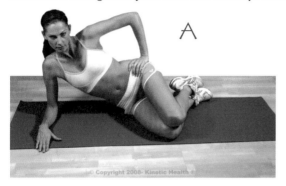

A

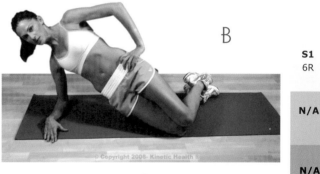

B

S1
6R

N/A

N/A

1. Lie on your side with your legs stretched out, and one arm bent parallel to the floor as shown in Image A.
   - Bend your knees to a 90-degree angle.
   - Brace your core and inhale.

2. Exhale as you lift your body up off the ground so that only your arm and knees are supporting the weight of your body.
   - Your body should form a straight line, from your head to your knees.
   - Do not allow your spine to curve forward or back.
   - Do not sag, and always continue to brace your core.
   - Distribute your body weight between your bent elbow and bent knees.

3. Hold the bridge for 10 seconds, then slowly lower yourself back to the ground.

4. Repeat the exercise for the recommended number of repetitions and sets, on both sides.

Front-to-Side Bridge

Front-to-Side Bridge - This advanced exercise is excellent for strengthening your core and improving your neuromuscular responses. The key is to keep your core braced throughout this routine **by bracing your rib cage to your pelvis**. Do not allow your core to bend as you roll from one shoulder to the next. The Front-to-Side Bridge is an advanced exercise that combines the movement patterns of both the front and side bridge, and acts to stabilize the shoulder, core, and lower extremity.

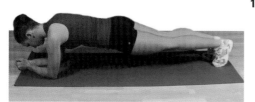

1. Starting position: Begin on the floor in the classic front bridge or plank position as shown in *Beginners Front Bridge - page 157*. Brace your core and inhale.

2. Turn your torso slightly so that you can lift your **right arm** into the air.

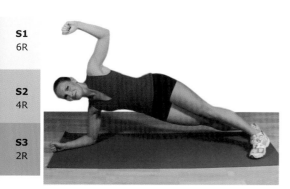

S1
6R

S2
4R

S3
2R

   - Slightly stagger your feet so you have a base of support while in this position.
   - Your upper body weight should be distributed on the left forearm.
   - Hold the side bridge position for two seconds.

3. Return to the starting front bridge position.

4. Repeat from step 1 for the opposite side, lifting your **left arm** up as you turn your torso and distribute your body weight onto the right side.

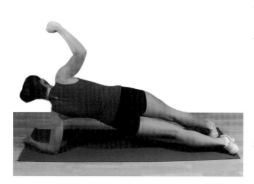

5. Repeat this sequence for the recommended number of repetitions and sets.

Russian Twist with Medicine Ball - This advanced exercise really works and strengthens the rectus abdominus and the external and internal oblique abdominal muscles. These muscles are involved in twisting motions such as those in golf, baseball, and racquet sports. The exercise and medicine balls add elements of proprioception and balance to your exercise.

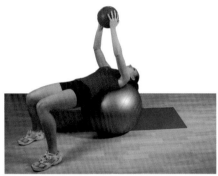

1. Starting Position:
   - Sit on a medium size exercise ball and hold a weighted medicine ball close to your chest with both hands.
   - Roll forward so that your back is resting comfortably on the exercise ball.
   - Keep your knees perpendicular to the ground, and your ankles and knees aligned.
   - Keeping a slight bend in your elbow, lift the medicine ball straight up, above your chin.

S1	S2	S3
10R	8R	6R

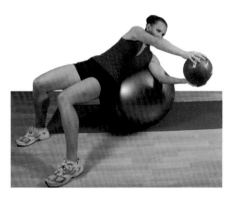

2. Brace your core and inhale as you twist your torso to the right for a count of two.

3. Roll back to the centre and then over to the other side for another count of two to compete this repetition.

4. Perform the recommended number of repetitions and sets.

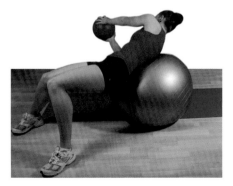

Draw a Sword - This exercise strengthens the muscles of the rotator cuff (supraspinatus, infraspinatus, subscapularis and teres minor). The rotator cuff plays an essential role in all actions that require internal or external rotation of the shoulder. This exercise should not cause pain. If you feel pain, reduce the tension in the tubing and try again.

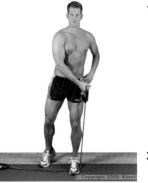

1. Stand on the tubing so that it is secure under your left foot, and cannot snap out.

   - The handle should be on the left side.
   - Reach across with your right hand and grasp the handle firmly, palm facing out, left hand on your hip.
   - Ensure you have sufficient tension. The tubing should not be floppy.
   - Brace your core and inhale.

2. Exhale, and pull the tubing diagonally out from your left hip, past your right hip, and up above your head as if you are drawing and brandishing a sword!

   - Keep your arm extended, but do not lock the elbows.
   - Maintain an upright posture.
   - The tubing should feel tight and stretched.

3. Hold the extended posture for a count of two.

4. Perform this exercise for the recommended number of repetitions and sets, for BOTH sides.

S1
10R

S2
8R

S3
6R

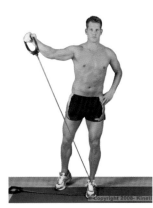

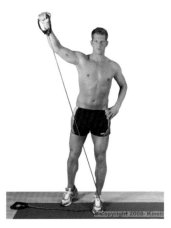

Throw a Javelin - This tubing exercise is great for strengthening the shoulders. It also acts to increase the motor connections between the upper extremities, core, hips, and lower extremities.

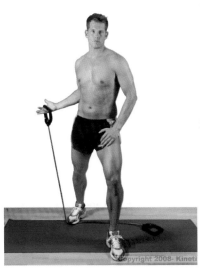

1. Start in a semi-lunge position, with the rubber tubing firmly under the back right foot, and the handle in your right hand.
   - The tubing should feel tight at hip level.
   - Palm facing upwards.

2. Pull your right hand up and forward, as if you are throwing a javelin.
   - Maintain your semi-lunge posture.
   - Hold the extended position for a count of two.

3. Perform this exercise for the recommended number of repetitions and sets, for BOTH sides.

S1
10R

S2
8R

S3
6R

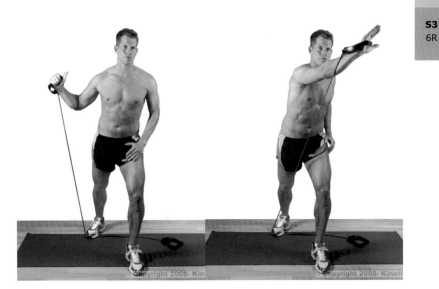

Medicine Ball Wood Chop - This dynamic exercise simulates the action involved in chopping wood. It develops core strength, improves speed and reaction time, and increases your neuromuscular control. This is a great exercise for improving your golf swing.

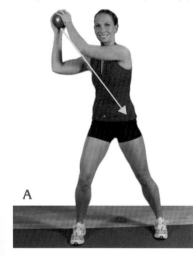

A

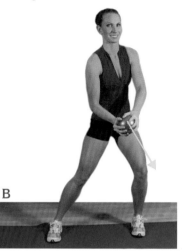

B

S1	12R
S2	10R
S3	8R

1. Hold a moderate weight or medicine ball in both hands.

2. Raise both hands to one side of your body as shown in Image A.

3. Pivot and bring the ball diagonally down towards the opposite knee.

4. Perform the entire sequence for the recommended number of sets and repetitions, for both sides.

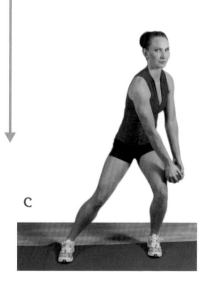

C

Performance Care for the Shoulder

Only use the remainder of these shoulder exercises if you are able to comfortably and easily perform the exercises in *Advanced Upper Arm and Shoulder Workout - page 82* and remain completely injury free. These advanced shoulder exercises integrate and use multiple elements of your shoulder's kinetic chain. See *Performance Care for the Arm to Shoulder - page 101* for more information.

- ❏ Advanced Alternating Dumbbell Press on Ball ....see page 166
- ❏ Single Leg Lateral Wood Chop ....see page 167
- ❏ Standing Lateral Raise ....see page 168
- ❏ Ball Transfer on the Floor ....see page 169
- ❏ V-Sit Medicine Ball Twist ....see page 170
- ❏ Kneeling Swiss Ball Rollout ....see page 171
- ❏ Swiss Ball Push-ups ....see page 172
- ❏ Single Hand Push-ups on Medicine Ball ....see page 173
- ❏ Push-ups with Unequal Hands ....see page 174
- ❏ Twisting Lunge on Medicine Ball ....see page 175
- ❏ Lunge with Medicine Ball ....see page 176
- ❏ Bridge on a Swiss Ball ....see page 177
- ❏ Side-to-Side Swiss Ball Hip Stretch ....see page 178

Advanced Alternating Dumbbell Press on Ball - This is
basically a dumbbell bench press, but by performing it on a ball with
alternating hands and feet, you are able to activate and use more of your
core and upper and lower extremities, while increasing your
neuromuscular control.

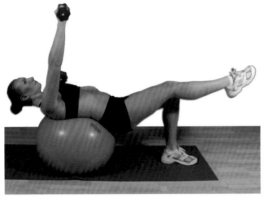

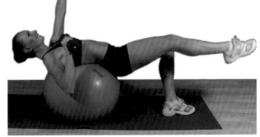

S1
12R

S2
10R

S3
8R

1. Starting position:
   Lie face-up on an
   exercise ball, back fully
   supported by the ball,
   and with the
   dumbbells by your
   shoulders.

   ■ Activate your scapula and keep it activated throughout the
     exercise. See *Setting and Activating the Scapula - page 118*.
   ■ Brace your core muscles (*How to Brace your Core! - page 24*).
   ■ Raise your right leg, while keeping your left foot firmly on the
     ground.

2. Raise the right dumbbell straight up above your shoulder for a count of
   two, keeping your back and shoulder flexed.

3. Return the right dumbbell to the starting position for a count of three,
   and repeat the procedure for the left dumbbell.

4. Reverse your leg position halfway through your set.

5. Perform the recommended number of sets and repetitions, alternating
   the leg position within each set.

Single Leg Lateral Wood Chop - This exercise combines lateral rotation with proprioception and balance. This is a great exercise for developing core power, and balance. This will help recruit more of your neuromuscular system and is a great golf performance exercise. Ensure the rubber tubing is firmly attached to an un-movable object (closed door, beam, etc.) before you start this exercise.

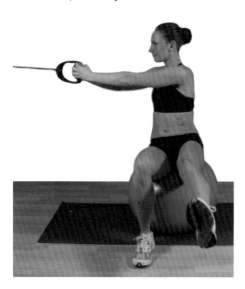

1. Sit on the exercise ball with both hands grasping the rubber tubing at shoulder level, on your *right* side.

2. Raise your *left leg* while maintaining your balance.

3. Pull the rubber tubing straight across your body to the left side while maintaining your balance.

4. Return to the starting position.

5. Repeat for the recommended number of sets and repetitions.

6. Then reverse sides and repeat for the opposite side.

S1	S2	S3
12R	10R	8R

Note: To increase the difficulty of this exercise, try alternating your legs with *each* repetition.

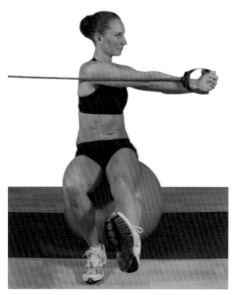

Standing Lateral Raise - Use this exercise to strengthen your rotator cuff muscles and build shoulder stability. This exercise is much more effective with weighted handballs since the gripping action activates more accessory muscles.

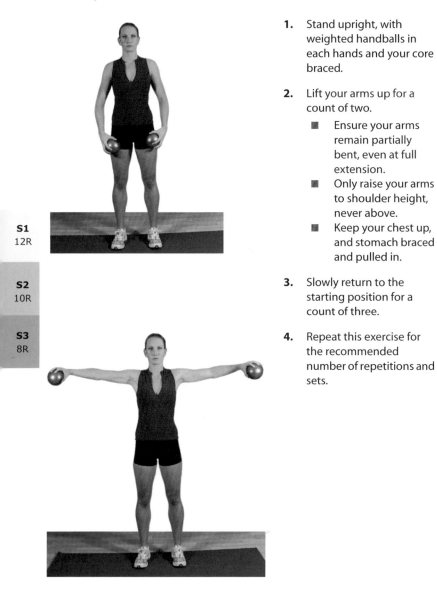

S1
12R

S2
10R

S3
8R

1. Stand upright, with weighted handballs in each hands and your core braced.

2. Lift your arms up for a count of two.
    - Ensure your arms remain partially bent, even at full extension.
    - Only raise your arms to shoulder height, never above.
    - Keep your chest up, and stomach braced and pulled in.

3. Slowly return to the starting position for a count of three.

4. Repeat this exercise for the recommended number of repetitions and sets.

Ball Transfer on the Floor - This is a fantastic exercise for building power and neuromuscular coordination between your core and extremities (arms and legs). Once you start this exercise, do not allow your hands or your feet to touch the ground. The goal is to keep your core activated throughout the exercise.

1. Lie on the floor, arms extended overhead, and an exercise ball grasped between your ankles as shown in image A. Squeeze the exercise ball between your ankles and raise your legs about five inches off the ground.

A

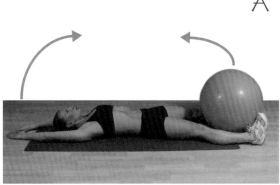

2. Tighten your abdominals and raise your legs to bring the ball towards your head. At the same time reach forward with your hands to grasp the ball halfway, as in image B.

3. Allow your arms to drop back above your head while holding the ball and at the same time return your legs to the starting position (5 inches above the ground).

4. Repeat this action in reverse to return to position A. This entire motion should be smooth and graceful.

B

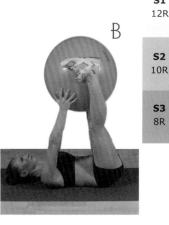

S1
12R

S2
10R

S3
8R

5. Repeat for the recommended number of sets and repetitions.

C

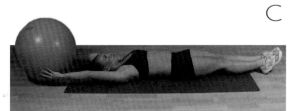

V-Sit Medicine Ball Twist - This exercise develops the stability of your lumbar spine while increasing abdominal strength by targeting one side of your abdominals at a time.

A

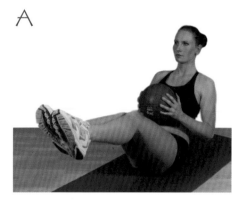

1. Starting Position: Hold a weighted medicine ball and lean back so that your body forms a V position as shown in image A.

2. Keeping the medicine ball stretched away from your body, twist to one side until the ball almost touches the ground.

B

3. Return to centre and repeat step 2 for the other side.

S1
12R

4. Repeat this sequence for the recommended number of sets and repetitions.

S2
10R

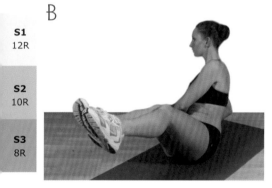

S3
8R

5. To make this exercise even more challenging, try the same exercise while sitting on a BOSU Balance Trainer or SitFit.

Note: Maintain a straight spine and keep your abdominal muscles contracted throughout the exercise.

C

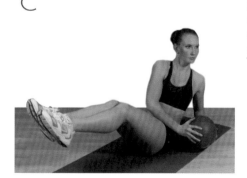

Kneeling Swiss Ball Rollout - This is a great exercise for developing general torso strength, improving pelvic control, and working your core, especially your abdominal muscles.

1. Starting Position: Kneel on a mat with the Swiss ball positioned in front of you, hands on the ball.

2. While maintaining contact with the ball, push it forward, tightening your core while maintaining a neutral spine.

3. Continue to push the ball as far as you can while still keeping your core tight, and your spine aligned.

4. Return to the starting position.

5. Repeat this exercise for the recommended number of sets and repetitions.

   - Be sure to do only as many repetitions as you can do while maintaining *perfect form*.

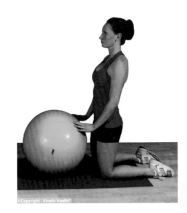

S1
10R

S2
8R

S3
6R

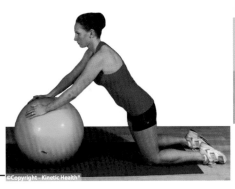

Note: To make this exercise more challenging, start the exercise in a Bridge position with straight legs.

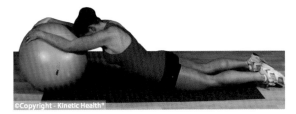

Swiss Ball Push-ups - This exercise combines the benefits of both push-ups and bridges. Your abdominals are strengthened since they are required to play a greater role in maintaining balance, stability, and proprioception.

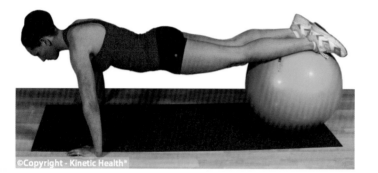

S1
12R

S2
10R

S3
8R

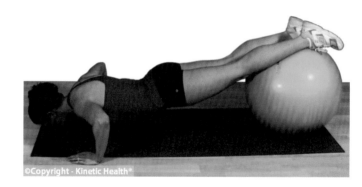

1. Starting position: Place both feet on a Swiss ball and your hands shoulder-width apart on the ground. Brace your core and keep your spine in neutral position.

2. Slowly lower your body down until your elbows are at 90 degrees, while keeping your body in a straight plank alignment.

3. Hold this position for a count of two.

4. Slowly push up to return to the starting position.

5. Repeat this exercise for the recommended number of sets and repetitions.

Single Hand Push-ups on Medicine Ball - This advanced push-up increases arm, upper body, and shoulder strength, while integrating proprioceptive actions to improve balance and challenge your neuromuscular coordination. You should feel its effects in your chest (pectorals), back of your arms (triceps), shoulders (deltoids), and rotator cuff muscles.

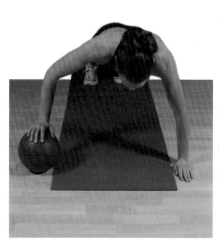

1. Starting position: Assume a stable plank position with an exercise ball under one hand.

2. Slowly lower your body down towards the ground, until your other elbow is bent at 90 degrees, while keeping your body in a straight plank alignment.

3. Hold this position for a count of two.

4. Slowly push up to return to the starting position.

5. Repeat this exercise for the recommended number of sets and repetitions, doing half the number of repetitions for one side and half for the other.

S1	10R
S2	8R
S3	6R

Note: The key to this exercise is to keep your core braced so your hips, core and shoulders remain in alignment. Be careful *not* to hinge at your waist.

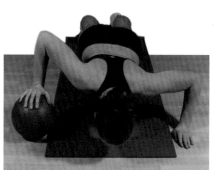

Push-ups with Unequal Hands - So, you have done all those other push-ups, and are finding them just a little too easy, and perhaps boring. Try this challenging version to really strengthen those muscles in your core and upper extremity. Do not perform this push-up until you are able to easily complete the exercises in the *Advanced Shoulder* routine.

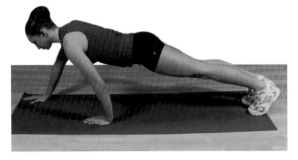

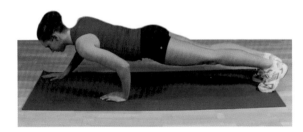

S1
12R

S2
10R

S3
8R

1. Starting Position:
   - Get into a standard push-up position.
   - Place your right hand parallel to, and beside your face.
   - Place your left hand beside your waist.
   - Play around with these hand positions to increase or decrease the level of difficulty.
   - Exhale, straighten your arms, and push *up* off the floor for a count of two.

2. Brace your core and hold the pushed-up position for a count of two, then lower yourself slowly to the ground for a count of three.

3. Rest for a count of one, and repeat from Step 2.

4. Repeat this exercise for the recommended number of sets and repetitions.

5. Then switch your arm positions and repeat for the opposite side, for the same number of repetitions and sets.

Twisting Lunge on Medicine Ball - This exercise strengthens your entire core, building power from your hips right up to the upper extremity. This exercise works your hamstrings, gluteals, quadriceps, hip flexors, core and shoulders. You will require a 5-12 lbs medicine ball for this exercise.

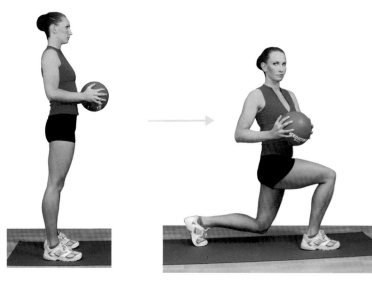

S1
12R

S2
10R

S3
8R

1. Starting position:
    - Begin in an upright standing position, spine in neutral position, holding a medicine ball with both hands.
    - Brace your core.

2. Step forward with one knee and drop down into a forward lunge position.
    - The front leg should form a 90-degree angle to the hips.
    - Do not allow the front knee to extend beyond your toes.
    - Keep the back knee an inch above the ground.

3. Twist your upper body toward the direction of the bent knee and hold for a count of two. Contract your back gluteal muscle while holding this position.

4. Stand and return to the neutral starting position.

5. Repeat for the recommended number of repetitions and sets, for both sides.

Lunge with Medicine Ball - This exercise works your entire kinetic chain, from your arms, through your core, and down your legs, while activating and improving the neuromuscular coordination and communication throughout your body. You will require a 5-to-12 lb medicine ball for this exercise.

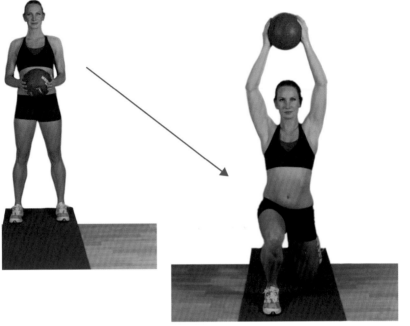

S1
12R

S2
10R

S3
8R

1. Starting position:
   - Begin in an upright standing position, spine in neutral position, holding a medicine ball, at waist level, with both hands.
   - Brace your core.

2. Step forward with one knee and drop down into a forward lunge position, while raising the medicine ball above your head at the same time.
   - Your chest should be in an upright position.
   - The front leg should form a 90-degree angle to the hips.
   - Do not allow the front knee to extend beyond your toes.
   - Keep the back knee an inch above the ground.

3. Stand and return to the neutral starting position.

4. Repeat for the recommended number of repetitions and sets, for both sides.

Bridge on a Swiss Ball - This exercise develops core strength in the muscles of your trunk, activates your kinetic chain, improves posture and alignment, and improves your balance and proprioception. Do not attempt this exercise until you can perform a normal bridge comfortably.

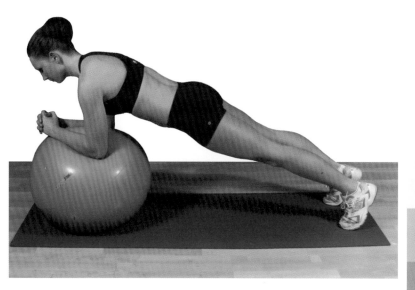

S1
10R

S2
8R

S3
6R

1. Starting position:
   - ■ Support yourself on the ball with your elbows, forearm, and toes.
   - ■ Brace your core.
   - ■ Be sure that your back is not hyper-extended, and that your legs, hips, core, shoulders, and neck are in alignment.

2. The key to this exercise is to maintain this ideal position. Only perform the number of repetitions that allow you to maintain this perfect form.

3. Hold this position for a maximum of 10 to 12 seconds.
   - ■ This exercise is used to develop stability.
   - ■ Holding this position for too long will put your muscles into an anaerobic state, which could be counter-productive when building a strong, solid base.

4. Repeat for the recommended number of repetitions and sets.

Side-to-Side Swiss Ball Hip Stretch - This is a great exercise for stretching your core, especially your spinal rotators.

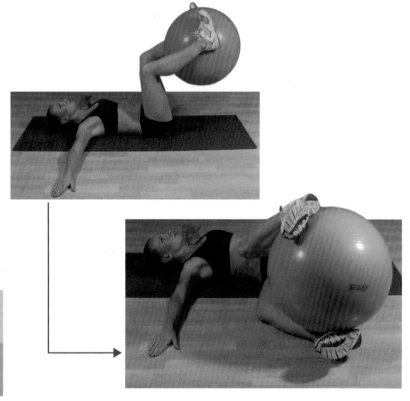

S1
12R

S2
10R

S3
8R

1. Starting position:
    - Lie on your back with a Swiss Ball between your legs.
    - Stretch your arms out to the side, keeping your shoulders on the ground.

2. Lift the ball up with your legs, knees bent to a 90 degree angle. Then slightly squeeze the ball with your heels and legs.

3. Twist your lower body to lower the ball to one side, and hold for a count of two. Make sure your knees do not touch the ground.

4. Now cross over to the other side, and repeat the same procedure. Crossing over from one side to the other counts as one repetition.

5. Repeat for the recommended number of repetitions and sets.

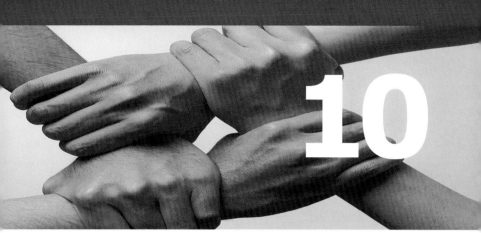

10

Exercises for the Hand and Wrist

Relaxing the Hand and Wrist

Stretches for the Hand and Wrist

Strengthening the Hand and Wrist

Massaging Trigger Points in Your Hand - Trigger points are
tender points in your muscles where you will find palpable nodules in tight
muscle fibres. These are areas where blood flow has decreased, lactic acid
has built up, and muscles have tightened up to form "knots" or "nodules"
of tissue.

There are two types of trigger points - **Active** and **Latent**. When you
compress an Active Trigger Point, it will refer pain to other areas of your
body. Compression of a Latent Trigger Point will only cause pain at the
point of compression, but will not refer pain. Trigger point massage
focuses upon releasing the tightness in these hyper-irritable sports.

All the trigger point massages in this book make use of a golf ball to apply
pressure upon the trigger point to release the restrictions. For each of the
following structures:

Apply Trigger Point Therapy

1. Roll the golf ball in firm, circular motions across the area for 10 to 20
    seconds.
2. When you find an area that is particularly tender, use the golf ball and work
    this area for an additional 20to 30 seconds until you feel a softening of the
    trigger point.
    - Monitor the level of pain on a scale of 1 to 10 (where 10 is excruciating
      pain). Do not exceed a level seven pain.
    - Ask yourself, "Would I be willing to do this again tomorrow?" If not,
      you are pressing too hard, so back off on the pressure.
    - Don't be aggressive with your therapy.
    - Be consistent with your therapy. Perform the trigger point therapy
      several times a day.

After Trigger Point Therapy

- Always drink several glasses of water.
- Walk around, or move the affected area to increase blood flow to the
  structure, and to keep your muscles warm, relaxed, and mobile.

Where to Apply Trigger Point Therapy for your Hands

For the purposes of this book, you can use a golf ball to apply pressure
upon the trigger points of your hands. Apply trigger point therapy as
shown on the following page, to these structures and their surrounding
tissues:

- thenar eminence muscles
- adductor pollicus muscle
- interosseous muscles
- hypothenar muscles
- palmar fascia

Massaging the Thenar Eminence Muscles - This area contains three major muscles: abductor pollicis brevis, flexor pollicis brevis, and the opponens pollicis. These muscles play an important role in any gripping action that is performed by your thumb.

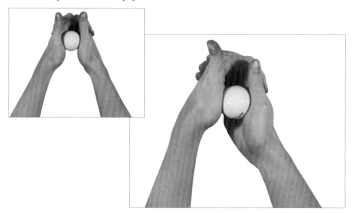

1. Interlace your fingers with the golf ball clasped between the thenar eminences.
2. Roll the golf ball **up** and **down** until you find a point of tension, and then perform small **circular motions** in that area to release the tension.

Massaging the Adductor pollicis - The adductor pollicis adducts the thumb (thumb opposition) and helps to flex the first thumb joint. It is commonly injured during gripping actions.

1. Place the back of your hand on your lap.
2. Roll the golf ball from the centre of your palm towards the base of your thumb, using small back-and-forth motions that follow the directions shown by the arrows in Image A.

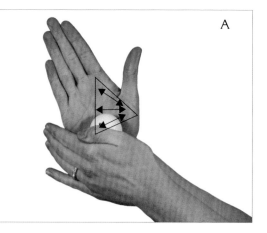

Working the First Dorsal Interosseous Muscle - The first dorsal interosseous muscle is often injured from repetitive actions such as keyboarding or writing. Injury to this muscle is often indicated by pain directly between your thumb and index finger, along the back of your hand. When this muscle is injured, you will have difficulty grasping objects between your thumb and index fingers.

1. Place your hand, palm down on your lap.

2. Roll the golf ball up and down from the web at the base of your thumb to the base of your index finger.

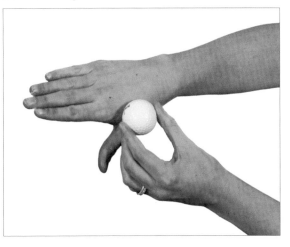

Massaging the hypothenar eminence muscles - The hypothenar eminence is made up of three muscles: abductor digiti minimi, flexor digiti minimi, and opponens digiti minimi. These muscles are often involved with ulnar nerve entrapment resulting in decreased grip strength and altered sensation to the 4th and 5th fingers.

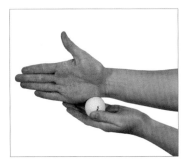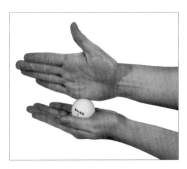

1. Cup the ball in one hand and roll it in an up-and-down motion across the hypothenar eminence muscles.

2. When you find an area of tenderness, use small circular motions to release the restrictions in that area.

Working the Palmar Fascia - The palmar fascia is a tough fibrous band of connective tissue covering the palm of your hand. If this fascia becomes thickened, it can cause the fingers to pull in towards the palm of the hand. This condition, known as Dupuytren's Contracture, occurs more frequently with smokers, diabetics, and people with cardiovascular conditions. Restrictions in the palmar fascia may inhibit opening and closing of the hand, and all associated gripping actions.

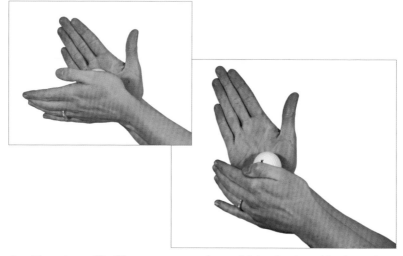

1.   Place the golf ball between your palms, roll it in a back-and-forth motion across the entire palmar fascia.

2.   When you find an area of tenderness, use small circular motions to release the restrictions in that area.

Tai Chi Chuan - Waking the Chi - Tai Chi Chuan is a Chinese Martial Art that aims to promote health and longevity. Chinese Martial Arts play considerable attention to flow, flexibility, strength, and even kinetic chain relationships. Injuries are reduced with this form by increasing the range of motion through dynamic stretching. The following exercise is typically done as a warm-up before starting a Tai Chi form. It works all your structures from your fingers to your shoulders.

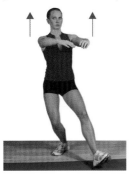

1. Stand with feet slightly apart, back foot flat on the ground, front heel down, toes pointing up.
   - Keep your head, neck, and back aligned in neutral position.
   - Keep your shoulders back and relaxed.
   - Keep your hips centred.

2. Inhale, and gently raise both your arms in front of your body, and then above your head for a count of five.

3. Turn your palms outwards to face the ceiling.

4. Exhale, and push your hands down your sides in a large circular arc until you reach your hips for a count of five.

5. As you do these motions, focus upon:
   - Executing the action slowly.
   - Breathing slowly and in rhythm with your actions.

6. Repeat this circular motion for the recommended number of repetitions and sets on each side.

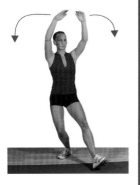

S1	10R Right
S2	10R Left
N/A	

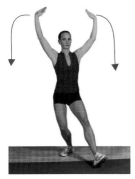

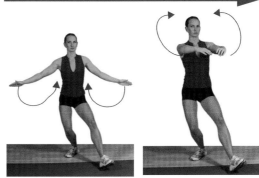

Tai Chi Chuan - Withdraw & Push - The following exercise is from the Yang style of Tai Chi. This sequence works all your structures from your fingers to your shoulders. When performed properly, you should feel blood flow from your fingertips to your shoulders, and your muscles should feel loose and relaxed.

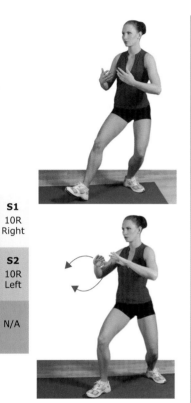

S1
10R
Right

S2
10R
Left

N/A

1. Stand with one foot ahead of the other, knees slightly bent.
   - Keep your head, neck, and back aligned in neutral position.
   - Keep your shoulders relaxed and back.
   - Keep your hips centred.

2. Gently raise your arms up to the level of your chest, as if you are holding a large ball.

3. Exhale, turn your palms outward, and push your hands outwards for a count of three. As you do these motions, focus upon:
   - Executing them slowly.
   - Breathing slowly and in rhythm with your actions.

4. When you reach the end-position, turn your palms inwards, inhale, and pull your hands back towards your chest for a count of three.

5. Repeat this circular motion for the recommended number of repetitions. Then change your leg position and repeat for the other side.

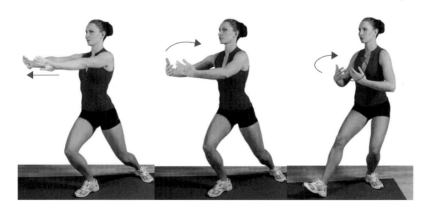

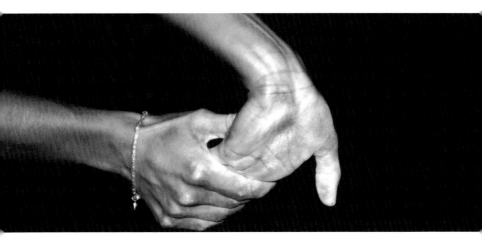

Stretches for the Hand and Wrist

Stop Right There - Forearm Extensor Stretch. Most people don't give their forearms a lot of attention (unlike their biceps and triceps). Forearms are pretty low maintenance, until you injure or stress them. But strong, limber forearms can help you to easily lift weights, swing that tennis racquet, or hit a golf ball further.

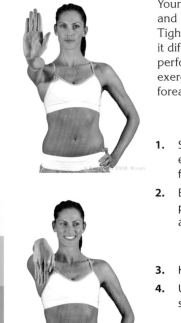

Your wrist extensors let you bend your wrist and hand towards the back of your forearm. Tightness and restrictions in this area make it difficult for you to use a keyboard, or perform actions such as writing. This exercise stretches the muscles in your forearm and wrist.

S1
5R
Right

S2
5R
Left

N/A

1. Stand in a relaxed posture with one arm extended straight in front of you, palm facing forward.

2. Bend your wrist downwards so that the palm of your hand is now facing your body, and your fingers point to the ground.
   - Do not let your shoulder rise up or hunch as you do this.

3. Hold this position for 10 seconds.

4. Use your other hand to gently pull your stretched hand towards your body.
   - Maintain your extended arm posture.
   - Keep your fingers over the knuckles of the bent hand.
   - You should feel a stretch along your entire wrist and upper forearm.

5. Hold this second pose for another 10 seconds.

6. Perform this exercise for **both hands** for the specified number of sets and intervals.

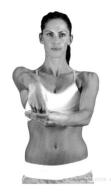

Variation - Repeat the first 3 steps, but make a fist before bending the wrist downwards.

Forearm Flexor Stretch - Your wrist flexors play an important role in any sport or activity involving gripping. This muscle group lets you bend your wrist and palm towards the front of your forearm. Tightness and restrictions in this area make it difficult for you to pick up or carry objects in your hand. Restrictions in these muscles often cause nerve entrapment syndromes.

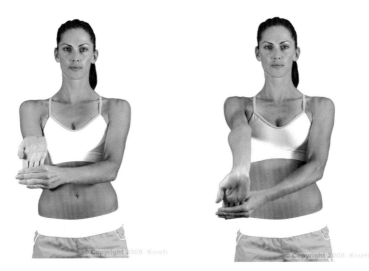

S1	30 sec
S2	25 sec
S3	20 sec

1. Stand in a relaxed posture with the affected arm extended in front of you, elbow slightly bent, with your palm facing up, and your fingers extending down towards the floor.

2. Place the fingers of your other hand over the inside of the knuckles, pull the extended hand back towards your body, and extend your elbow.
   - Maintain your extended arm posture.
   - You should feel a stretch along your entire wrist and inner forearm.

3. Hold this pose for 20 to 30 seconds.

4. Perform this exercise for **both hands** for the specified number of sets and intervals.

Variation - Repeat the first 3 steps, but make a fist before bending the wrist downwards.

Note: If you have tingling or numbness down the length of your forearm, you can use a variation of this stretch to floss your nerves. Perform the same exercise, but tuck your chin down into your chest as you extend your elbow.

Subscapularis Wall Stretch - This wonderful exercise stretches many of the major muscles of the shoulder and upper arm including the triceps, subscapularis, serratus anterior, teres minor, and teres major.

The subscapularis muscle is often tight and restricted when you have a shoulder injury. This muscle is used in backhand strokes in tennis and other racquet sports, as well as in the front crawl in swimming. When this muscle is injured, you may find it difficult to sleep on your side, or be unable to raise your arm overhead.

S1
20
sec

S2
20
sec

S3
20
sec

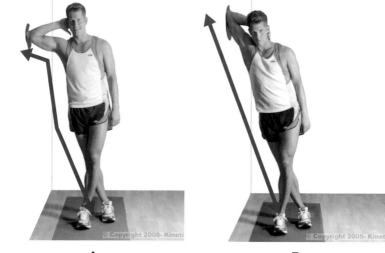

A   B

1. Move into your starting posture:
   - Place your feet about two feet from the wall.
   - Cross your right leg over your left as shown in Image A.
   - Lean your elbow against the wall.
   - At this point, your body should be relaxed with no tension or strain.

2. **Exhale** as you lean your hips into the wall.
   - Increase the stretch by leaning your upper body towards the wall.
   - Your body should form a straight line from elbow to ankle as shown in Image B.

3. Perform this exercise on **both sides** for the specified number of sets and intervals.

Attention: Avoid slumping or dropping your head forward when you perform this exercise.

Namaste - This classical prayer position improves your shoulder posture while stretching your fingers, wrist, and forearms.

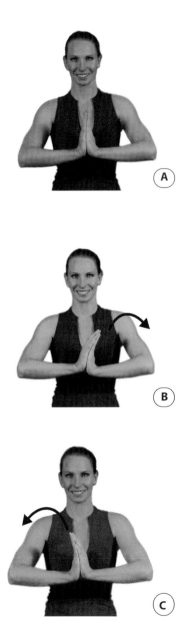

1. Sit with your spine in neutral position, with good posture, and your scapulae activated. See Massage Your Neck and Shoulders ....see page 110.

2. Adopt the classic prayer or "**Namaste**" position, as shown in image A.
   - Push your palm and fingers firmly together.
   - Raise your elbows so that your forearms are parallel to the floor.
   - Ideally your wrist should form a right angle with your arm and hand, while your forearms remain parallel to the floor.

3. Push your hands together while maintaining proper elbow alignment and shoulder position.
   - Hold this pose for 10 seconds.

4. Now use the tips of your fingers to alternately push and flex-extend the tips of your fingers back and forth, while maintaining your starting posture. See Images B and C.

5. Repeat this waving flexion-extension for the recommended number of repetitions and sets.

S1
7R

S2
6R

S3
5R

Waiter's Tip – Nerve Flossing Exercise - Dr. Michael Leahy first showed me this exercise for stretching and translating the radial, median, and ulnar nerves as they pass through the surrounding soft-tissue structures. This exercise acts to break the adhesions that tether the nerves to surrounding tissues, that inhibit the normal translation of nerves through the tissues, and which can result in a variety of nerve compression syndromes.

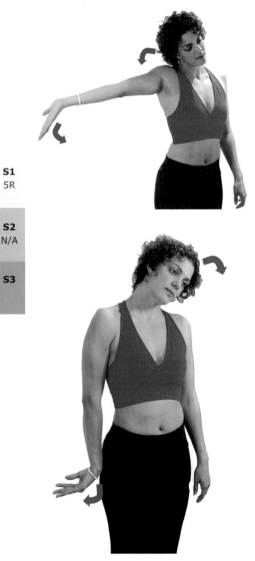

S1
5R

S2
N/A

S3

1. Part 1: Stand in a relaxed posture with the right arm extended to the side, parallel to the floor, palm facing up.

2. Extend your wrist to stretch the fingers of your hand towards the floor.

   - Keep the upper arm level with the shoulder.
   - Keep the other shoulder relaxed.

3. Part 2: Bring your right ear to your shoulder with no rotation and hold the stretch for a count of eight (8).

4. Now, drop your right arm down to your side, rotate your arm in with your palm facing up. This position is like a waiter waiting for his secret tip.

   - Bend your head towards the left side – ear to shoulder with no rotation.
   - Hold for a count of eight.

5. Repeat this exercise for the specified numbers of sets and repetitions, for both sides.

Floss your Median Nerve - Just like flossing your teeth, you can floss your nerve and keep it from getting jammed (due to adhesion formation) between tissue layers. The median nerve runs down the arm and forearm, and passes through the carpal tunnel. When the nerve is trapped or restricted, you will feel numbness, tingling, and loss of function in your first three fingers. This exercise stretches and helps to release and translate the median nerve across all the soft-tissue structures through which it passes. This is a great stretch if you have Carpal Tunnel Syndrome.

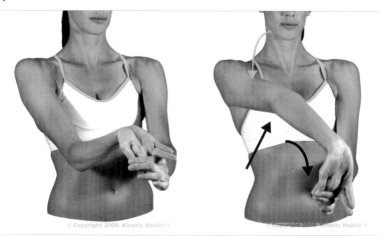

S1
30S

S2
30S

S3
30S

1. Extend the right arm in front of your body, palm facing up.

2. With the other hand, grasp the middle, index, and thumb fingers of the right hand.

3. With the palm facing away from you, pull your fingers towards your body until you feel a strong stretch.
   ■ Hold this stretch for 30 seconds to stretch and release the median nerve.

4. You can increase the nerve translation by tipping your head down and slightly towards your shoulder as you stretch your fingers.

5. Repeat this stretch for the specified number of sets for each hand.

Note: For cases of Carpal Tunnel Syndrome, you can perform this stretch once every hour, throughout the course of each day.

Floss your Radial Nerve

Floss your Radial Nerve - The radial nerve innervates the extensor muscles of your triceps, the back of your forearm, and the extensors of your hand.   The radial nerve passes through a tunnel of muscles and bone at your elbow, and if it is trapped or restricted, you will feel pain and tenderness on the outside of your elbow, with symptoms similar to tennis elbow. This exercise stretches and helps to release and translate the radial nerve across all the soft-tissue structures through which it passes.

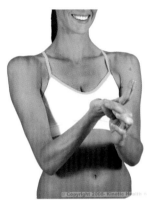
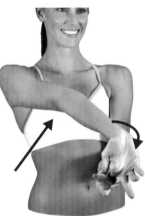

S1
30S

S2
30S

S3
30S

1. Extend the right arm in front of your body, palm facing up.
2. With the other hand, grasp the index finger and thumb of the right hand.
3. With the palm facing away from you, pull these two fingers towards your body until you feel a strong stretch.
   - Very gently, twist your fingers slightly toward the thumb for a full stretch.
   - Hold this stretch for 30 seconds to stretch and release the radial nerve.
   - Release the stretch when you feel a decrease in the tension of your hand.
4. Increase nerve translation by tipping your head forward, and slightly towards your shoulder as you stretch your fingers.
5. Repeat this stretch specified number of sets for each hand.

Attention: If your radial nerve is severely entrapped (or adhesed to surrounding tissues) you may need to first release the entrapments through treatments such as Active Release Techniques.

Floss your Ulnar Nerve - When your ulnar nerve is entrapped or restricted, you will find that you have limited ability to use your hand to perform daily functions. Restrictions to the ulnar nerve frequently occur at the Guyon Tunnel in the wrist, and in the Cubital Tunnel near the elbow and can result in tingling down your ring and little fingers. This exercise stretches and helps to translate and release the ulnar nerves across all the soft-tissue structures through which it passes.

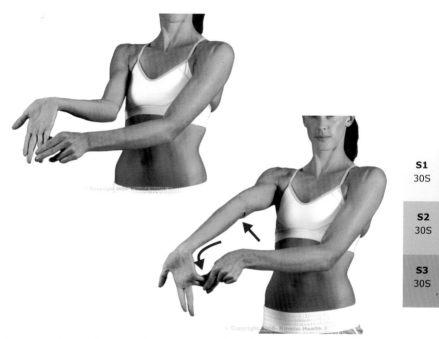

S1
30S

S2
30S

S3
30S

1. Extend the right arm in front of your body, palm facing up.
2. With the other hand, grasp the ring finger and little finger of the right hand.
3. With the palm facing away from you, pull these two fingers towards your body until you feel a strong stretch.
    - Hold this stretch for 30 seconds to stretch and release the ulnar nerve.
    - Release the stretch when you feel a decrease in the tension of your hand.
4. Increase the flexion by tipping your head forward and slightly towards your shoulder as you stretch your fingers.
5. Repeat this stretch for specified number of sets for each hand.

Strengthening the Hand and Wrist

One Hand Grip Strength

One Hand Grip Strength - This exercise strengthens the muscles of the hand. You will need to use a Power Web for this exercise. Power Webs are used to rehabilitate and strengthen the muscles of your fingers, wrist, and forearm.

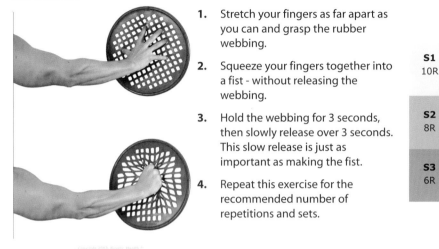

1. Stretch your fingers as far apart as you can and grasp the rubber webbing.

2. Squeeze your fingers together into a fist - without releasing the webbing.

3. Hold the webbing for 3 seconds, then slowly release over 3 seconds. This slow release is just as important as making the fist.

4. Repeat this exercise for the recommended number of repetitions and sets.

S1
10R

S2
8R

S3
6R

Two Hand Grip Strength

Two Hand Grip Strength - This exercise strengthens the muscles of the hand, and the forearm extensors and flexors. Your goal is to stretch the Power Web EQUALLY with both hands.

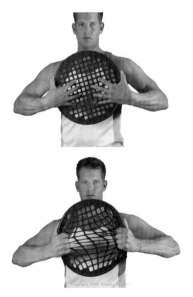

1. With both hands, grasp the centre of the power web.

2. Pull the power web with both hands towards its outer edges as shown in this image. Try to keep the expansion balanced for both hands.

3. Hold the webbing in this position for 3 seconds then slowly release over 3 seconds.

4. Repeat this exercise for the recommended number of repetitions and sets.

S1
10R

S2
8R

S3
6R

One Hand Grip with a Twist - This exercise strengthens the muscles of the hand, especially those involved in supination and pronation. You will need to use a Power Web for this exercise. Power Webs are used to rehabilitate and strengthen the muscles of your fingers, wrist, and forearm.

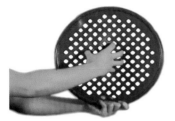

1. Stretch your fingers as far apart as you can and grasp the rubber webbing. The wider you stretch your fingers, the greater the resistance provided by this exercise.

2. Squeeze your fingers together into a fist - without releasing the webbing.

3. Twist the webbing by turning your wrist.

4. Hold the webbing for 3 seconds, then slowly release over 3 seconds. This slow release is just as important as making the fist.

5. Repeat this exercise for the recommended number of repetitions and sets.

6. Repeat this sequence but twist in the opposite direction.

S1
10R

S2
8R

S3
6R

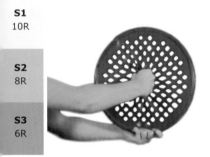

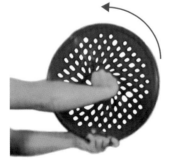

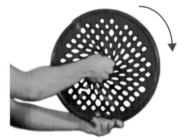

Handball – Wrist Inward Curl

Handball – Wrist Inward Curl - The only way to increase the strength of your wrist is by increasing the strength of the hands and forearms. This exercise combines the benefits of gripping exercises with forearm strengthening. This exercise trains the pronator teres, flexor carpi radialis, palmaris longus, flexor carpi ulnaris, and flexor digitorum superficialis muscles. You will need a soft handball that is large enough to prevent your fingers from encircling the ball. This larger size ball will help to build strength in your fingers and thumbs, as well as develop muscle strength in your forearms. We recommend you start with a 2-to-4 lb. weight. Alternatively, use any free-weight that you have available.

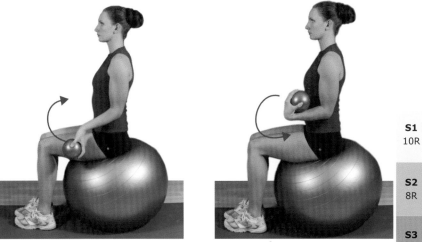

S1
10R

S2
8R

S3
6R

1. Sit on an exercise ball, with your elbow bent to 90°.

2. Firmly grasp the soft handball in your hand, with your palm facing **upwards**.
    - Allow your wrist to drop down as shown in image A.
    - Select a handball weight with which you can comfortably flex your wrist, starting with 2 to 4 pounds.

3. Bend your wrist upwards (palm up) for a count of three, as far as possible.
    - Hold the flexed position for three seconds.
    - Maintain a firm grip on the handball. This allows you to activate more muscles in your forearm.

4. Maintaining a firm grip, lower the handball slowly for a count of three, keeping your forearm parallel to your thigh.

5. Repeat this exercise for the recommended number of repetitions and sets, for *each* hand.

Handball – Wrist Lift (extension) - If you spend long hours in front of a computer, your wrist and forearm extensors can become tight, restricted, and weak. This wrist extensor exercise will help to extend the muscles of your forearm, while combining the benefits of gripping exercises. This exercise works the extensor carpi radialis, extensor carpi radialis brevis, extensor carpi ulnaris, and extensor digitorum muscles.

You will need a soft handball which is large enough to prevent your fingers from encircling the ball. This larger size ball will help to build strength in your fingers and thumbs, as well as develop muscle strength in your forearms.

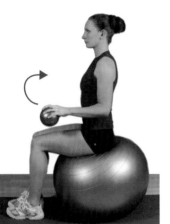 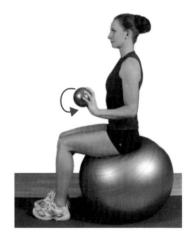

S1
10R

S2
8R

S3
6R

1. Sit on an exercise ball, with your arm bent to 90°.

2. Firmly grasp the soft handball in your hand.
   - Allow your wrist to drop down over your knee as shown in image A, with your palm facing **downwards**.
   - Select a handball weight with which you can comfortably flex your wrist, starting with a 2-to-4 pound weight.

3. Extend your wrist upwards (palm outwards) for a count of three, as far as possible.
   - Maintain a firm grip on the handball. This allows you to activate more of the forearm extensor muscles.

4. Lower the ball slowly for a count of three, keeping your forearm level to your thigh.
   - Continue to maintain a firm grip on the ball.

5. Repeat this exercise for the recommended number of repetitions and sets, for *each* hand.

Lift a Beer - Now it's time for some serious training....Oktoberfest anyone? But, instead of a beer can, we would like you to use a soft-weighted handball (2 to 4 pounds) to perform this exercise.

This exercise strengthens and increases the ability of the abductor pollicis longus, flexor carpi radialis, extensor carpi radialis longus, and extensor carpi radialis brevis muscles to radially deviate, while strengthening your fingers and thumb at the same time.

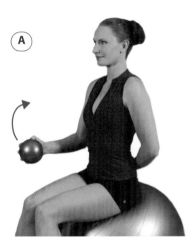

A

1. Sit on an exercise ball, with your elbow bent to 90°, handball in your hand, palm facing inwards as shown in image A.

2. Flex your wrist **upwards** (thumb up) as far as possible, keeping the palm facing inwards. See Image B.
   - Hold the flexed position for 3 to 5 seconds.
   - Maintain a firm grip on the soft exercise ball.

3. Lower the ball slowly for a count of three, keeping your forearm level to your thigh as in image C.

4. Repeat this exercise for *each* hands for the recommended number of repetitions and sets.

S1
10R

S2
8R

S3
6R

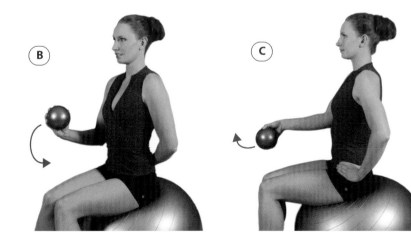

B

C

Handball - Twist the Doorknob - In this exercise, you will use your grasping and turning actions to strengthen the muscles involved in pronation and supination of your wrist and forearm. **Pronation**, in which your forearm rotates to place your palm face down, is performed by the pronator quadratus and pronator teres muscles. **Supination**, in which your forearm rotates to place your palm face up, is performed by your biceps brachii and supinator muscles.

S1
10R

S2
8R

S3
6R

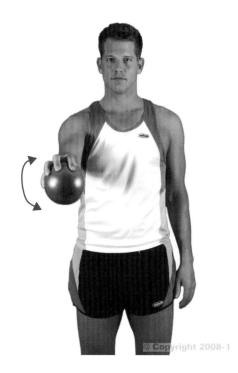

© Copyright 2008- 1

1. Sit or stand comfortably, with your affected hand grasping an exercise handball.

2. Extend the affected hand in front of you, below shoulder height, arm slightly bent.

3. Firmly grasp an exercise handball in your hand, and twist your wrist from left to right and back again, as if you are turning a door knob.
   - Ensure you maintain a firm grip on your handball.
   - Select a handball weight with which you can comfortably rotate your wrist.

4. Repeat this exercise for the recommended number of repetitions and sets, for *each* hand.

Building Hand Dexterity

Building Hand Dexterity - This hand dexterity exercise takes your hand through unfamiliar motions to improve its flexibility and definition.

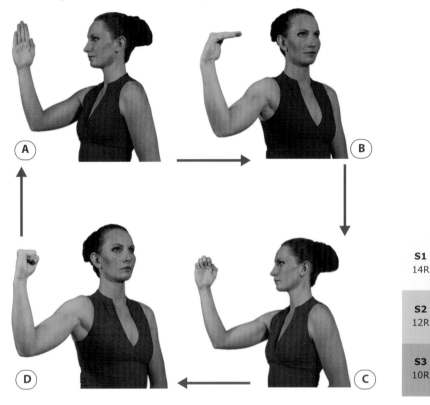

S1
14R

S2
12R

S3
10R

1. **Starting Position**: Place your hand in front of you, fingers together, as in Image A.

2. Bend all four fingers downwards to form a right-angle with your palm. Keep your fingers straight, and do not change the position of your thumb. See Image B.

3. Now push your fingers back to form the right-angle at your first finger joint, again maintaining your thumb position. See Image C.

4. Now roll your fingers down into a tight fist, with your thumb overlaying all the fingers. See Image D.

5. Now *reverse these actions* to return to your starting position.

6. Repeat this exercise for the recommended number of repetitions and sets, for *both* hands. With practice, these actions should become smooth and elegant, rather than jerky and stiff.

Golf Ball Roll - Proprioception, strength, and endurance exercise for your fingers. This exercise increases your hand's proprioception, coordination, and strength. You will need two golf balls to do this exercise.

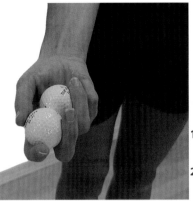

S1
60
sec

S2
50S
sec

S3
40
sec

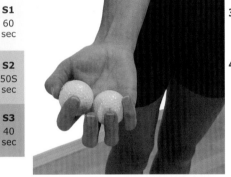

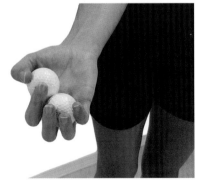

1. With your arm extended, hold the two golf balls in your hand.

2. Using your fingers, rotate the two balls in a clockwise direction. Do this for 60 seconds.

3. Now reverse the motion of the balls in a counter-clockwise direction. Do this for 60 seconds.

4. Repeat this exercise for the recommended number of repetitions and sets, for *both* hands.

Bharatnatyam Finger Dexterity - Indian classical dance requires a great deal of dexterity and strength in the hands and fingers. To achieve this goal, this ancient dance form has developed a complex series of gestures that all students must learn. I found it useful to teach them this little exercise to warm-up their hands and increase their strength.

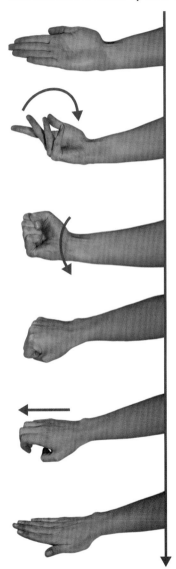

1. Extend both hands in front of your body, palms facing up, fingers stretched out.

2. Starting with your little finger, fold each finger into your palm, ending with your thumb on top of your folded fingers to make a fist.

3. Maintaining your fist, *flip your hand over*, keeping your arms out stretched.

4. Now SLOWLY unwrap your fingers, pushing your kinetic energy through the fingertips.

5. Return to your starting position.

6. Repeat this exercise for the recommended number of repetitions and sets, for *both* hands. After a while, these actions should become smooth and elegant, rather than jerky and stiff.

7. As your dexterity improves, try the following:
   - Increase the speed of movement.
   - Reverse the direction in which you touch fingers to palm.

S1
14R

S2
12R

S3
10R

Isometric Finger Touch - Believe it or not, finger injuries happen often, but rarely receive much attention. Given how much we do with our fingers, it is well worth your time to do some basic finger dexterity and strengthening exercises on a daily basis. This is another great exercise for dancers, musicians, keyboard operators, writers, and students.

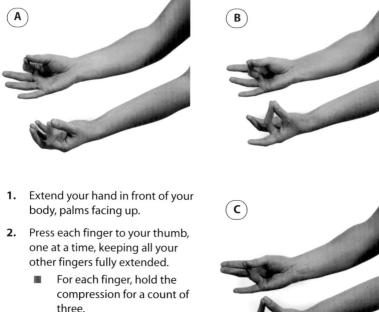

S1
14R

S2
12R

S3
10R

1. Extend your hand in front of your body, palms facing up.

2. Press each finger to your thumb, one at a time, keeping all your other fingers fully extended.
   - For each finger, hold the compression for a count of three.

3. Repeat this exercise for the recommended number of repetitions and sets, for *both* hands.

4. As your dexterity improves, try the following:
   - Do both hands at once.
   - Increase the speed and pressure of movement.
   - Reverse the direction in which you touch thumb to finger.

Finger Wave - Our kids were in drama class and showed us this finger dexterity exercise. They do it so fast that all you can see is a continuous waving blur. But we will start a little slower. Try this fun little exercise to keep your fingers flexible, fast, and agile.

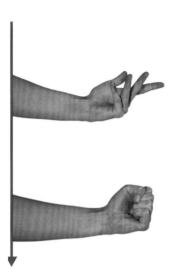

1. Extend both hands in front of your body, palms facing upwards.

2. Starting with your left hand - make a waving double fist:
   - Close your LEFT thumb into your palm.
   - Repeat with each subsequent finger.
   - Transfer to the right hand and close your little finger into your palm.
   - Repeat with each subsequent finger till you reach your RIGHT thumb.

3. Open your fists by starting with your right hand:
   - Open and extend your RIGHT thumb.
   - Repeat with each subsequent finger.
   - Transfer to the left hand and open and extend your LEFT little finger into your palm.
   - Repeat with each subsequent finger till you reach your LEFT thumb.

4. Repeat this exercise 10 to15 times in a smooth continuous motion going from left to right, and back again from right to left, like a wave passing from one hand to the other.

5. Increase your speed as your dexterity improves.

S1
10R

S2
8R

S3
6R

Finger Joint Rotations - This exercise improves the rotational capabilities of each individual finger (three joints per finger). Each joint is surrounded by a joint capsule that can become fibrotic, and inhibit joint movement. This is especially true with arthritic conditions. This exercise can often restore mobility to arthritic joints or prevent arthritic joints from developing.

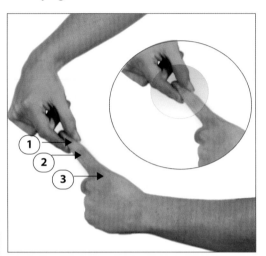

S1
10R

S2
8R

S3
6R

1. Surround the end joint of the finger with the index finger and thumb of the other hand.

2. Make a firm contact and rotate the joint clockwise, then counter-clockwise, while at the same time slightly tractioning the finger (pull your finger).

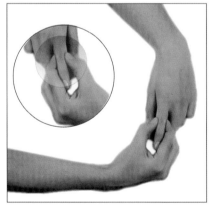

3. Perform this back and forth rotation 10 times.

4. Then change your position on the same joint and repeat for another 10 times.

5. Perform this exercise on all three joints of each finger.

6. Repeat this exercise for each finger for the recommended number of sets and repetitions.

Gyroscopic Strengthening

Gyroscopic Strengthening - This remarkable little gyroscopic-powered ball uses gyroscopic resistive power to work up your arm's entire kinetic chain, strengthening your wrists, forearms, and shoulder. It also aids in developing neuromuscular control of the entire upper extremity. This is a wonderful exercise for climbers, racquet sports players, golfers, and swimmers.

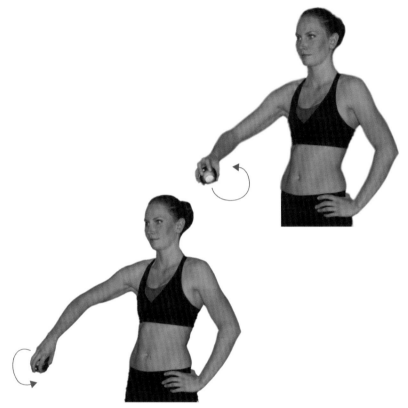

1. Hold the gyroscopic-ball in your right hand, and extend your arm out as shown in these images.
2. Rotate your wrist in a circular motion to activate the gyroscope.
3. Perform a clockwise rotations for 30 to 60 seconds.
4. Then reverse the direction for another 30 to 60 seconds.
5. Perform this exercise for each hand for approximately two to five minutes.

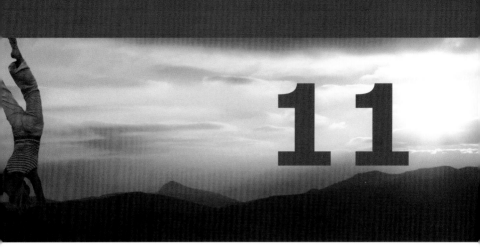

Self Care Tips and Hints

Since soft-tissue and joint injuries are very common, it is good to know what you can do to take care of yourself when it happens. Rapid treatment is essential for ensuring quick recovery from these injuries.

The tips and hints we are providing in this chapter relate to the care of sprain/strain or minor joint injuries that occur due to repetitive actions, trauma, poor body mechanics, inflammation, excessive stress to the muscles and tissues of your body, and muscle imbalances within your kinetic chain. They do not apply to serious trauma or emergency situations.

Note: In this book, we are **not** talking about dealing with traumatic injuries involving open wounds, bleeding, impaled objects, extreme force injuries, etc. For such cases, seek immediate care from your medical practitioner.

For most non-traumatic soft tissue injuries, start self-care with the following:

- ■ **Cold Therapy** ....see page 212.
- ■ **Heat Therapy** ....see page 214.
- ■ **Epsom Salt Baths** ....see page 216.
- ■ **Benefits of Rest** ....see page 217.
- ■ **Exercise** ....see page 218.

Cold Therapy

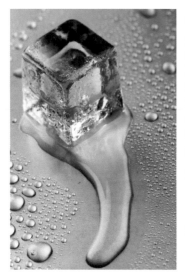

When you have a soft-tissue injury, you will often feel pain and muscle spasms. Your area of injury may become inflamed and swollen due to the tearing of blood vessels and the release of fluids into the damaged area. Your first goal in treating most soft-tissue injuries should be to:

- Slow the release of hormones and chemicals that cause the pain and inflammation.

- Reduce inflammation by decreasing the movement of fluids into the area.

The easiest and most effective means to do this is **Cold Therapy**. Cold therapy helps numb the nerves, reduce pain signals being sent to the brain, reduce muscle spasms, reduce swelling by constricting the blood vessels, reduce cell death by decreasing the rate of metabolism, and reduce blood flow to the area.

Cold therapy should be the FIRST treatment for inflammation! And...it should be applied within the first 48 hours of injury–the sooner, the better. In many cases, applying ice within the first hour can reduce healing times by as much as 50%.

Yes, we know that HEAT sounds much more tempting and comforting – especially when you are in pain or are living in colder climates. But, remember that heat therapy increases blood flow to an area, and therefore can cause more inflammation and pain... something you want to avoid during the acute stages of inflammation!

Tips and Hints for Icing

- While icing, elevate the injured area – preferably above the heart – to reduce swelling by moving blood away from the affected area.

- Ice every two to three hours, but first make sure that the area being iced has warmed up and is no longer numb.

- Prevent frostbite by not allowing the ice pack to sit directly on your skin. Use a thin towel in-between.

When Not to Ice!

Do not use Cold Therapy if the person:

- Is unconscious, unable to communicate, or has no sensation in the injured area.

- Tends to develop a rash or blisters when exposed to cold.

- Has circulatory problems.

- Has Raynaud's disease, rheumatoid or gouty arthritis, kidney malfunctions, or hyperthyroidism.

Icing with an Ice-Pack

- Place a thin cloth on the injured area.
- Apply the ice-pack to the injured area.
- Keep the ice-pack against the affected area until it feels numb.

You should first feel **cold**, then a **burning sensation**, followed by **aching**, then **numbness**. If you don't feel numb, then you haven't iced for long enough.

- This process takes about 15 to 20 minutes. Never longer!
- Do NOT allow the skin to freeze...you are not trying to get frost-bite.
- Leave a minimum of one hour between each icing session to allow your tissues to warm up.

Ice Massage

Ice massage can be more effective than regular icing.

- Fill small paper cups with water and keep them in your freezer till frozen.
- Peel the top of the cup back to expose the ice.
- Massage the ice over the injured area in small circular motions, allowing the ice to melt away.
- Use a towel to catch the melting water.
- To **prevent tissue damage**, only perform ice massage for a maximum of 7 to 9 minutes.

Heat Therapy

Without a doubt, Heat Therapy feels much nicer and more comforting than Cold Therapy. But problems can arise when heat therapy is used too soon after an injury or trauma. In fact, the early use of heat therapy by our patients is often the primary reason for the increased time required to resolve their soft-tissue injuries.

Heat Therapy should only be used *after inflammation has subsided.* Never use heat therapy within the first 72 hours of an acute injury. Applying heat to soft tissues (muscles, ligaments, and tendons) while the area is still inflamed and swollen will only aggravate the injured tissues. During the first 72 hours, cold therapy provides much more effective and appropriate relief.

Benefits of Heat Therapy

Once the inflammation has subsided, you can apply heat to the affected area to help restore flexibility, relieve muscle cramping, reduce arthritic symptoms, and most of all, to increase the rate of healing by increasing blood-flow to the area.

The power of heat therapy comes from its depth of penetration and its ability to increase circulatory and neurological function. Increasing circulation results in increased delivery of oxygen and nutrients to the affected area while at the same time displacing waste by-products. Heat affects the nervous system by stimulating the sensory receptors in your skin. This has the effect of decreasing the transmission of pain signals to your brain, thereby reducing muscle spasms and episodes of acute pain.

Types of Heat Therapy

The effectiveness of heat therapy varies from individual to individual. Each person needs to experiment to determine which therapy is best suited to their condition. There are two primary types of heat therapy:

- **Moist Heat**: Moist heat therapy includes hot baths, heated whirlpools, hot packs, or hot moist towels. Many people feel they get better depth of penetration with moist heat.

- **Dry heat**: Dry heat therapy includes dry saunas, electric heating pads, and heat lamps. These can be very effective forms of heat therapy but they also tend to dehydrate the individual, so remember to drink lots of fluids when you use dry heat therapy.

For how long should you apply heat therapy? For a minor, superficial injury you may only want to use heat therapy for 10 to 20 minutes. For chronic injuries, you may need to apply heat therapy for 20 to 35 minutes.

Heat Treatment with a Hot Towel

- Dampen an old, clean towel (towels may discolour with this process).
- Heat the moist towel in a microwave for one to two minutes. Check the temperature of the towel, and heat for another minute if necessary.
- Carefully remove the moist hot towel (don't give yourself a steam burn) and wrap the hot towel with a dry towel (to prevent burns, and to retain the heat).
- Apply the hot towel to the affected area until your muscles relax and warm up, and your skin turns slightly rosy.
- Stop after 15 to 20 minutes. Do not re-apply for at least 1 to 2 hours.

Attention: Always use caution with Heat Therapy. Use only moderate heat to avoid burning the soft tissue. Do not use heat treatment if you suffer from one or more of the following conditions: cancer, diabetes mellitus, tendency to hemorrhage, decreased sensations, peripheral vascular disease, acute inflammation, cognitive impairment, deep vein thrombosis, dermatitis, heart disease, hypertension (high blood pressure), skin lesions, or open wounds. If in doubt, consult your physician!
Try to avoid using Heat Therapy at night, or when you are in bed. You are more likely to fall asleep with the heating pad, and that could be dangerous since it can cause burns and overheating.

Epsom Salt Baths

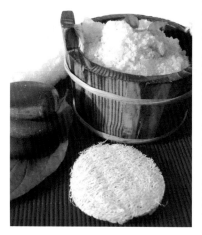

Grandmother's magic home remedy for aches and pains...epsom salts. Soaking in an epsom salt bath is one of the best things you can (and should) do for your body.

Epsom salts (magnesium sulfate) have a high concentration of magnesium, which help to draw out inflammation – pushing chemicals and toxins out of muscles and joints, relaxing muscles, and moisturizing skin.

But, remember that epsom salt baths is another form of Heat Therapy, and therefore all the rules that apply to Heat Therapy also apply to epsom salt baths.

After long runs, a hot bath with epsom salts is recommended to reduce the pain in aching legs. We recommend soaking in an epsom salt bath at least once a week to reduce daily aches and pains. You can also use epsom salts for reducing inflammation from localized soft-tissue injuries.

Using Epsom Salts Locally

- Fill a bucket of hot water, add one cup of epsom salts, and soak your sore feet or hands.
- Dip a wash cloth in epsom-salt-drenched water, and wrap it around your sore achilles tendon to reduce inflammation.
- Soak a cloth in epsom salt water, wring it out, and place it over a sore or painful area. Now wrap a tensor bandage or towel around everything to keep the heat in, and to hold the epsom-salt-soaked towel in place! It works wonders!

Make an Epsom Salt Bath:

Mix two (2) cups of epsom salts in lots of hot water.

Soak in the bath and let the Epsom Salts do their magic!

Benefits of Rest

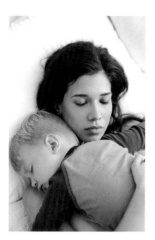

Rest, in our busy world, is becoming an increasingly rare commodity. But it is an essential component for healing your body.

Your body needs rest and sleep in order to function properly and to repair itself. While you sleep, your body performs much of its maintenance and renewal functions.

If you have any type of soft-tissue injury (caused by sports, career, home care, or just daily activities), you must *rest* that area to give it a chance to recover properly.

Lack of sleep results in decreased immune function, increased potential for disease (heart disease, stroke, cancer), decreased hormone production (human growth hormone), decreased tissue repair, decreased cognitive function, decreased fat metabolism, depression, increased inflammation, and even decreased life span.

Some very interesting research has come out of the National Academy of Science about the effects of sleep deprivation. Sleep deprivation causes an elevated level of the stress hormone, corticosterone. Increased levels of this hormone causes a reduction in the function of brain cells. This, in turn, has been directly related to problems in concentration and other possible cognitive issues. A little sad, but lack of sleep may even reduce cognitive function so much that you don't even realize there is a problem.

We have found that our patients' lack of rest and sleep is one of the primary reasons for a slow or delayed recovery from an injury. Avoid over-using an injured area before it is recovered as that can cause further injury, more inflammation, and increased healing time.

How much sleep you require will vary based on several factors, including your diet (good diet, bad diet), environmental factors (smoking, drinking), quality of sleep, genetics, and current injuries. Even the quality of light that you are exposed to will affect the amount of sleep you need (spending a long time in front of your computer disrupts your circadian rhythm). In general terms we recommend at least 7 to 8 hours of sleep per night.

Reducing sleep by as little as one-and-a-half hours for just one night reduces daytime alertness by about one-third. Bottom line: without proper sleep, your body will not repair itself, you decrease the overall quality of your life, and you may even decrease your life span.

So, immediately after an acute injury, reduce the activity performed by that structure, do *not* perform weight-bearing exercises that can stress that area, do apply Cold Therapy, rest that structure, and keep it elevated to reduce inflammation.

By doing these simple steps, you provide your body with a critical element needed for self-healing...REST!

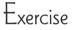

Exercise

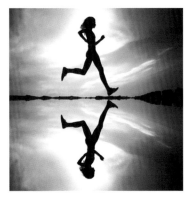

We have already talked about the importance of exercise in all aspects of your life.

When you have finished resting, icing, compressing, and elevating your injury, and once your inflammation has come down, you may want to start a moderate exercise program to get your damaged tissues back in gear.

This book, and its partners, show you how you can rehabilitate your tissues, and get back to an active lifestyle. Always start with the beginner's exercises to loosen those tight muscles and tissues, and as you progress, increase the intensity and type of exercise.

Remember, listen to your body...it is your best instructor and will tell you when you are overdoing things! So good luck...and get healthy and strong today!

Check our website at www.releaseyourbody.com for more information:

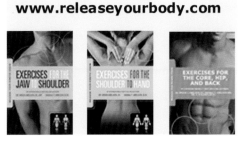

Release Your Kinetic Chain - Exercise Books

- Exercises for the Jaw to Shoulder
- Exercises for the Shoulder to Hand
- Exercises for the Back, Core, and Hip
- Exercises for the Hip to Toes

Release Your Pain – Resolving Repetitive Strain Injuries with Active Release Techniques

12

Alternative Therapies to Explore

The following section describes some of the types of practitioners with whom you might consider consulting when you have a soft-tissue injury that requires more assistance than exercise routines can provide. In all cases, to find the best practitioner, remember to check their certification and, where possible, ask for personal referrals.

Active Release Techniques® (ART)

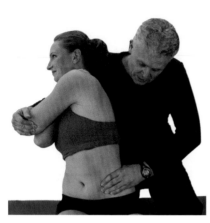

Dr. Abelson performing ART.

Active Release Techniques (ART) is, in my opinion, one of the **most** effective and reliable methods for releasing adhesions or restrictions between soft tissue layers.

Just about any soft-tissue injury can be treated effectively with ART. This technique has helped Olympic athletes, PGA golfers, professional hockey players, and football players win numerous events.

This multidisciplinary technique was developed by a Chiropractor, Dr. P. Michael Leahy of Colorado Springs, Colorado.

Essentially, ART is a hands-on soft-tissue technique that can simultaneously locate and break up scar tissue. The power of ART lies in how it combines patient motion with practitioner techniques to release the adhesions between tissue layers. This process restores mobility and relative motion to the soft tissue layers, increases circulatory function, and increases neurological function by breaking restrictive adhesions.

Effectiveness of Active Release Techniques

ART is at the top of my list for soft-tissue techniques, especially when it is performed correctly by a skilled practitioner. The key word is *skilled*! ART practitioners claim to have a 90% success rate, and this is quite true when the practitioner is both skilled and experienced. The key is to find someone with both the training and experience you require.

As I mentioned, I strongly recommend Active Release Techniques® for the treatment and resolution of a broad range of soft-tissue injuries. But due to its growing popularity and effectiveness, there are many people claiming to be ART practitioners, who have **not** received the required training.

It is very important to check out the certification levels of your selected ART practitioner. ART practitioners can take courses in Upper Extremity, Lower Extremity, Spine, Long Nerve Entrapment, and Biomechanics. Make sure your practitioner is certified for treating the areas that you require. In addition (as one of the writers of the *ART Online Biomechanics Course*), I can tell you that it is well worth your time and health to find someone who is also certified in *both* biomechanics and ART. These specialized individuals will be better able to find and identify exactly which restrictions are inhibiting your performance, and then help you to eliminate the problem!

To verify your ART practitioner's qualifications, visit the Active Release website at **www.activerelease.com**. This site tracks all current ART practitioners, and provides information about their current level of certification.

Note: If you are searching by geographical area, you may need to click SEARCH several times, since this database will only display a limited number of doctors for each search. If you live in an area with many ART practitioners, the system may only display only ten at a time. So click several times to see all the ART practitioners in your area.

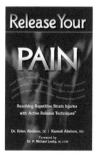

For more information about **Active Release Techniques**, you can also visit our websites at:

- www.activerelease.ca
- www.kinetichealth.ca.

In addition, to learn how ART can help resolve your soft tissue injury, you may want to read our best-selling book, **Release Your Pain** – *Resolving Repetitive Strain Injuries with Active Release Techniques*.

Visit www.releaseyourbody.com for more details.

Graston Techniques®

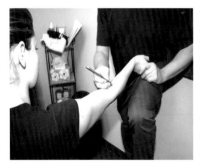

Graston Techniques® is an instrument-assisted, soft-tissue mobilization technique. The technique was initially designed by an athlete who suffered a debilitating knee injury.

Graston Techniques employs a combination of six hand-held, stainless steel instruments to release soft tissue restrictions.

The Graston instruments are used to separate and break down scar tissue (collagen cross-links). This process increases circulatory function and helps the practitioner to mobilize, reduce, and re-organize fibrotic restrictions in the neuromuscular-skeletal system.

As with other soft-tissue techniques, the practitioner must be skilled in the application and use of these instruments since considerable bruising can occur if this therapy is applied in too aggressive a manner.

The Graston tools can be of great benefit to many practitioners whose own joints and muscles suffer from Repetitive Strain Injuries (RSI). As a patient, this means your practitioner can use these tools to access severely restricted areas in your body, without causing further repetitive strain injuries to their own hands and body!

Graston Techniques® was first researched at Ball Memorial Hospital and Ball State University at Munci, Indiana. Today, there are more than 3000 clinicians—including Athletic Trainers, Chiropractors, Physiotherapists, and Occupational Therapists—who use Graston Techniques.

Effectiveness of Graston Techniques

In my opinion the power of this technique lies in its use as an adjunct – therapy, one which is best combined with other soft tissue modalities.

I believe this is especially true when the practitioner is dealing with nerve entrapment syndromes where he or she needs to find the location of the nerve, and release it from surrounding adhesed tissue, but must move through many layers of adhesed, entrapped soft tissue layers to do so.

Graston Techniques can be highly effective, especially when used in conjunction with other hands-on techniques such as Active Release Techniques, Manipulation, and Massage Therapy. However, after having applied both this and other soft-tissue techniques, I must say that there is nothing that matches the tactile sensitivity and effectiveness of a skilled practitioner's hands.

Note: With Graston Techniques it is common to experience some discomfort during the procedure, and find some minor bruising afterwards. This is usually nothing to worry about as it is just part of the normal healing process.

For more information, see www.grastontechnique.com.

Manipulation

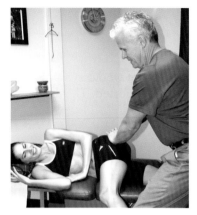

Dr. Abelson performing a Chiropractic manipulation.

Manipulation is used to treat musculoskeletal conditions, to relieve pain, and to improve neuromuscular function by restoring freedom to both spinal and peripheral joint movement.

In addition, through the effective manipulation of the spinal column and the body's extremities, there can be a substantial improvement in nervous system function.

Historical records show that manipulative therapies have existed for thousands of years. Manipulation has been documented in Chinese and Indian literature as far back as 2000 years ago. In China, manipulation has always been considered an effective form of therapy. This statement holds more weight when you consider that these Chinese physicians were only paid when their patients remained healthy. Now that is what I call a proactive health care system.

Today the most common types of western manipulation are Chiropractic and Osteopathic Manipulation. Both professions have a colourful history with no lack of controversy. The key point here is that all that controversy is historical! Today these medical professions are regulated by government bodies with strict criteria. Practitioners of both professions have no less than 7 years of post-secondary education. In fact, the first three years of their training is identical to any other medical professional.

Essentially, practitioners of manipulation move joints in a manner that frees up or breaks restrictions that are causing neurological or biomechanical problems. These biomechanical problems do not just include the joints themselves; manipulation also has a significant effect upon the body's soft tissues.

Manipulation affects muscles by causing the stress receptors in the muscles (Golgi tendons) to temporarily inhibit all activity in the areas being adjusted. This reaction causes the muscle group in the surrounding joints to go into an instantaneous state of relaxation. This intervention is a very important effect when your practitioner is trying to break a pain cycle. This approach to manipulation is strongly supported by scientific studies.

There are some opponents to manipulation that would still have the public believing that these therapies are unsupported. This is complete nonsense since there are literally hundreds of peer-reviewed scientific articles proving and supporting the benefits of manipulation.

Effectiveness of Manipulation

Manipulation is generally very safe and effective when performed by a trained professional. Just remember that manipulation can be used to treat musculoskeletal conditions, relieve pain, and improve function. I have seen hundreds of patient cases which would never have been resolved without manipulative treatments. On the other hand, for manipulation to remain effective, treatments must be combined with appropriate exercise. When manipulation is combined with soft-tissue techniques (such as Active Release Techniques, Graston Techniques, or Massage Therapy) it becomes even more effective since both joint and soft-tissue restrictions are removed or released.

Note: Unfortunately, some practitioners of manipulation get caught up in the marketing of their practices, rather than in achieving results. You may want to be a little concerned with practitioners who want to sign you up for a full year's worth of treatments!

Fortunately, this is not true for the majority of practitioners. The majority of practitioners are caring individuals who try to do the best they can for their patients. Good practitioners are going to try for the best resolution of your condition within the shortest time possible. The practitioner should provide you with a time frame for your treatment. For example, at our clinic this is usually 2 to 6 weeks (six weeks for severe cases). The practitioner should also provide you with specific exercises and other lifestyle recommendations that apply to your condition!

Massage Therapy

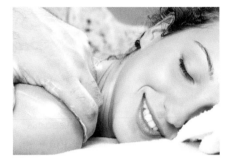

Massage is one of the oldest forms of touch-based healing. It can be used as a means of relaxation, or, in its deep-tissue form, to release restricted tissues.

Massage is not just an effective approach to pain management and rehabilitation, it also has tremendous physical, biochemical, and psychological benefits.

Massage increases circulatory function, increases blood oxygen levels, moves nutrients to needed areas, and displaces waste by-products. In fact, in terms of pain relief, some studies have shown that massage surpasses the effectiveness of numerous medications, without any of the negative side-effects.

Massage therapy has consistently been shown to help patients in dealing with their pain. This includes common muscle and joint pain as well as stress and pain arising from pregnancy, osteoarthritis, rheumatoid arthritis, and even cancer.

Massage therapy also provides huge psychological benefits in its ability to decrease stress and anxiety. Even stressed premature babies notice the difference. On the average, premature babies who receive regular massages gain 47% more weight than those who do not receive massage.

Effectiveness of Massage

Massage Therapy is very safe and highly recommended. Trained Registered Massage Therapists are very effective at treating and providing relief for a wide range of conditions such as migraine headaches, tendonitis, arthritis, osteoporosis, fibromyalgia, sports injuries, and a broad range of other common soft-tissue conditions. At Kinetic Health, we have several highly skilled therapists who work with us by combining their treatments with our own to help us achieve optimum patient results.

Finding a Massage Therapist

Since there are literally hundreds of different modalities that could be labeled as massage, there is no single governing body for the regulation of massage therapy. When you look for a Registered Massage Therapist, check for the following:

- Does the therapist have any experience in dealing with your particular type of soft-tissue injury?

- Does the Registered Massage Therapist have at least 1000 hours of training?

- How long has the Massage Therapist been practising?

- Is the Massage Therapist licensed?

- Who is the licensing authority and are they a reliable resource?

- Where did the Massage Therapist receive training?

- Does the Massage Therapist have any training in advanced or specific massage techniques?

- Can the therapist provide any supporting references?

Physiotherapy / Occupational Therapy

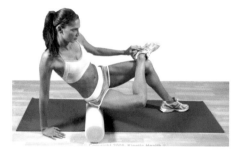

Physiotherapists and Occupational therapists are professionals who aim to rehabilitate and improve the condition of people who suffer from movement disorders.

To achieve their results, both professions use a combination of:

- Therapeutic exercises.
- Electrotherapeutic and mechanical agents such as ultrasound, TENS, short wave diathermy, interferential, ice, and heat.
- Functional training and some manipulation of joints and soft tissue.

Many of these therapists also take additional training in other techniques such as Acupuncture, IMS (Intermuscular Stimulation), Active Release Techniques, Graston Techniques, as well as a wide array of other procedures.

I teach courses with some great Physical and Occupational Therapists who I highly recommend. These individuals usually are very hands-on in their treatment approaches and provide their patients with individualized programs. They can truly be great resources of information. As a patient you could greatly benefit from this type of practitioner.

Effectiveness of Physiotherapy & Occupational Therapy

The effectiveness of Physiotherapy and Occupational Therapy, like many other professions, will vary greatly depending upon the practitioner's experience, skill, and the type of protocols that they implement. It is very important to find out from your potential therapist:

- What experience does the therapist have in treating your particular condition?
- How long will it take to resolve your condition?
- What type of results can you expect to receive from this treatment?
- Is the therapist licensed? With whom?
- Who is the Governing Body for this therapist?

It is also important to check on your therapist's current certification (via the local government body), especially where it applies to his or her additional training. For example, if a physiotherapist claims to be certified in acupuncture, check to see how much training they have actually received. Skilled Acupuncturists often have over 3000 hours of training, but many Physiotherapists (and Chiropractors) have less than 100 hours of training (not nearly enough, in my opinion).

You may also want to check if they are trained in areas such as Active Release Techniques or Graston Techniques. If yes, make sure their certification is current. When it comes to spinal manipulation, I would stick to a Chiropractor or Osteopath since a few weekend courses simply does not compare to four years of manipulative training.

Physiotherapists in Canada and the United States are required to register with a provincial or state governing body, with additional voluntary membership with a national association.

- If you are in Canada, visit **www.physiotherapy.com** for more information.
- If you are in the United States, visit **www.apta.org** for more information.
- For all other countries, please check with your state, provincial, or national organizations.

Acupuncture and Traditional Chinese Medicine

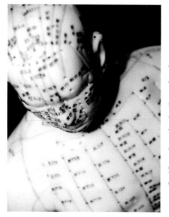

Acupuncture and Oriental Medicine are two of the fastest growing health care professions in North America.

Today, Doctoral training programs for Traditional Chinese Medicine (TCM) often provide an extensive curriculum which focuses upon both TCM and Western science. Performed correctly with great expertise, this can be a great tool for resolving many conditions.

For example, my younger sister, who suffered from partial paralysis after a stroke, regained full function within a short period of time due to treatments with acupuncture and oriental medicine. This is a great example how Chinese medicine can help resolve many conditions with which western medicine has had very limited success.

Western medicine is only just beginning to understand how these procedures actually work. Initially, many western doctors put the results down to the *placebo* effect. This attitude changed after studies by the Harvard Medical School using MRI brain imaging. Researchers using Functional Magnetic Resonance Imaging (fMRI) performed brain scans on normal subjects to investigate how Acupuncture affects brain activity.

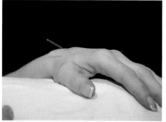

Acupuncture needle in the He Gu point.

All of the subjects had acupuncture needles inserted in the LI 4 (large intestine or He Gu point – located on the hand between the thumb and forefinger). In Acupuncture this point can be used to provide general pain relief during labour. Western medicine blew off this idea because there was no neurological or anatomical basis for this concept.

That was, of course, until they started testing the procedure with MRI brain mapping methodology. They found that the insertion and manipulation of the acupuncture needles at this point caused a pronounced calming of activity in many deep structures of the brain (amygdala, hippocampus, hypothalamus, etc.) accompanied by increased signal intensity in a key sensory region of the brain's cortex. There was only one conclusion that researchers could come to:

"Acupuncture regulates multiple physiological systems and achieves diverse therapeutic effects!"

Effectiveness of Acupuncture and Traditional Chinese Medicine

TCM can be very effective in the hands of a skilled practitioner. If you decide to seek out this treatment option, make sure you do your research and find out:

- Is your therapist certified in the technique?
- How many hours of training has he/she received?
- What experience does the therapist have in treating your particular condition?
- How long will it take to resolve your condition?
- What type of results can you expect to receive from this treatment?
- Is the therapist Board-certified and insured? With whom?
- Who is the Governing Body for this therapist? You should also be able to contact their local governing body to check on current certification.

As with all other Traditional Chinese Medicine techniques, these TCM procedures must be accompanied with appropriate exercise protocols. If a practitioner tells you that all you need is the TCM therapy and no exercise, then you should consider finding another practitioner.

INDEX **13**

INDEX

Acknowledgements and Thanks

This book is dedicated to our parents, without whose support, inspiration, and love, we would not be who we are today! Thanks so much Mom and Dad - on both sides!

This book would not have come into existence without the participation of some wonderful people - our office staff, patients, family, and friends.We would like to take this opportunity to thank each and every one of you for your support and patience as we underwent the long, arduous, and sometimes frustrating process of writing this four-volume set of books! **Thank you, Thank you**, all of you! In particular, we would like to thank the following for their time, participation, and talent!

Our fantastic sports models - Jenny Fletcher, Arlynd Fletcher, Miki Waters, Sherry Sands, and Corrine Lloyd. Your knowledge, technical expertise, time, and friendship made these photos a pleasure to take, and a pleasure to use! You are beautiful - inside and out!

Our patient and thorough editors - Dr. Tarveen Ahluwalia, Hannah MacLeod, and Kristin Meidal. Wow, when my eyes got blurry, and my brain just couldn't process anymore, you were there to catch all those bugs, nits, commas, and funny little words I just couldn't see anymore! Thanks so much.

Our talented graphic artists - Our special thanks to Lavanya Balasubramanian for her superb illustrations and photography skills. You are without a doubt one of the most talented and artistic people in our life. Your grasp of our needs, and your ability to make our visions come true is phenomenal, and your sparkling energy and joy in life make you a delight to work with. Thanks also to Kirk Oulette for his beautiful cover designs and for bringing a fresh new look to our book covers.

Biographies

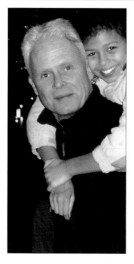

Dr. Brian Abelson DC - Brian's incredible, interdisciplinary knowledge of anatomy, physiology, human biomechanics, kinetic chain relationships, and exercise made these books possible. Just ask any of his patients, and they will fill your head with exclamations about how he can somehow *bring it all together* to solve their soft-tissue problems! And he brought it all together as we worked to design the exercise routines in these books...somehow integrating self-help exercises with his knowledge of soft-tissue restrictions, kinetic chains, and biomechanics to produce a graduated series of exercises that can help all of us to heal, recover, and perform at our best! Brian is a highly proficient Active Release Techniques Instructor and practitioner, trained in Graston Techniques, Chiropractic, Acupuncture and Chinese Medicine, Homeopathy, and Nutrition. He brings an integrated approach to health care which is very much appreciated by all his patients.

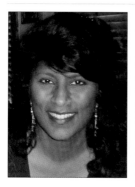

Kamali T. Abelson BSc - Kamali's long experience in the technical communication and publishing industry (25+ years) definitely came in handy as we wrote these books. Especially as they grew from the original vision of a 50-page booklet, into a four-volume set of books, each over 250 pages, packed with new illustrations, photos, and exercises.   She enjoys the company of her friends, being a mom and wife, running, hiking, travelling, dancing, and the arts. Given the opportunity, she would be spending most of her time travelling to distant corners of the world, taking dance and art lessons, meeting new people, and absorbing new cultures, thoughts, and ways!

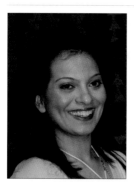

Dr. Tarveen Ahluwalia DC, BSc - Tarveen's medical and exercise knowledge combined with her friendship, enthusiastic participation, and technical edits helped to mold and develop these books. Tarveen is currently a Doctor of Chiropractic and Office Manager at Kinetic Health. She holds a Bachelor of Science in Kinesiology and is a certified Personal Trainer, and is a provider of Active Release and Graston Techniques. She enjoys time with her family and friends, speaking about health and fitness-related topics, and loves World music, weight training, running, hiking, travelling, cooking, reading, and Bhangra dancing.

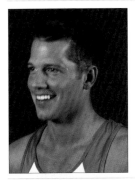

Arlynd Fletcher - Male model extraordinaire, with an amazing eye for positioning, light, and balancing photo shoots, all accompanied by a brilliant smile. Arlynd is also an incredible photographer in his own right! Brian and I bless the day we met you and Jenny.

Your help, professionalism, and ability to adjust the lighting to get just the right effect was priceless as we struggled to learn how to take exercise photos properly! You are awesome! Thanks so much for your help.

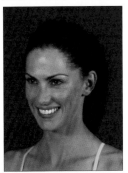

Jenny Fletcher - Supermodel Jenny Fletcher is incredibly photogenic and is also an amazing athlete. Every one of her exercise photos came out great. Today, Jenny is winning triathlons (*placing 1st in the 2009 Escape for Alcatraz*), appearing on the cover of sports magazines, and living an incredibly full life.

Read more about Jenny at www.jennyfletcher.com. It's been a privilege and pleasure watching you grow! Thanks so much for helping to make these books a reality.

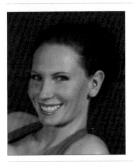

Miki Waters - Amazing massage therapist, great friend, and talented model...what more could you ask for! Oh yes...beautiful, too. Miki has been invaluable in getting our exercise vision onto paper. Her ability to hold a pose, even when the exercise leaves her quivering, is just another example of her professionalism...in all aspects of life!

Miki...it has been a pleasure working with you, getting to know you, and having you for a friend.

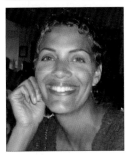

Sherry Sands - Massage therapist, wonderful friend, and a fountain of information. This multi-talented lady has been a part of our life for many years, and has modelled for both our international best-seller **Release Your Pain**, as well as other articles and publications.

She now works as a Production Accountant in the Calgary Oil Industry (did I say...multi-talented).

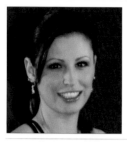

Corrine Lloyd - Another of our multi-talented, registered massage therapists, Corrine brought her brilliant smile, knowledge, and willingness to work hard at any exercise to all our photoshoots. Her joy in life brought exuberance and energy to all our sessions. You can see her in our books, brochures, and articles.

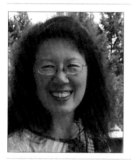

Lavanya Balasubramanian - This young lady brings sparkle and energy to our group...and never fails to lift our spirits. She is without a doubt one of the most talented artists we have ever met, and is able to take Brian's unique visions and present them artistically for our use, and your view. Her passion for our world, art, humanity, and the environment are a model for all of us! Here's to your continued growth...may you always sparkle bright!

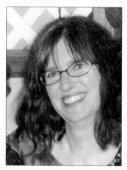

Hannah MacLeod - Wow...what a lady! Hannah has the most amazing eye for detail, and without her professional edits, and attention to all the details of presentation and content, this book would not be with you today. Of all our friends, Hannah has the most diverse set of hobbies and interests - from massage therapy and golfing, to knitting, spinning fibre, weaving, crafting, dancing, health, travel, and family! Love your YURTS, lady!

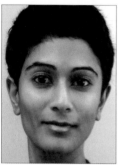

Kristin Meidal - Our long-time friend and co-worker. Kristin has a great eye for detail and pattern, and has helped throughout our writing process in ensuring consistency and clarity. Thanks again, Kris, for all that hard work; it's always a pleasure to work with you.

Publications from Kinetic Health

Written by the internationally best-selling authors of **Release Your Pain,** these books and exercise routines can help you release your pain, rehabilitate injuries, and help you achieve your best in both sports and daily life.

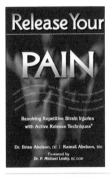

Release Your Pain - Resolving Repetitive Strain Injuries with Active Release Techniques
by Dr. Brian Abelson and Kamali T. Abelson

This international best seller has helped thousands of people resolve pain caused by repetitive strain and soft-tissue injuries, and is a great introduction to how the highly effective soft-tissue treatment method - Active Release Techniques - can help you recover from your soft-tissue injuries.
Available Now!

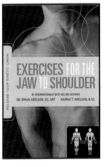

Exercises for the Jaw to Shoulder - Release Your Kinetic Chain by Dr. Brian Abelson and Kamali T. Abelson

If you suffer from headaches, jaw pain, TMJ, chronic neck pain, whiplash injuries, rotator cuff pain, shoulder pain, or other soft-tissue injuries of the jaw, neck, or shoulder, then this book may be exactly what you need. Instead of working with just the area of injury, these routines work with the Kinetic Chain, and can help you to take a key step towards resolving long-standing soft-tissue injuries and neuromuscular problems.
Available Now!

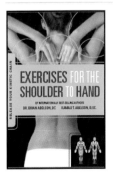

Exercises for the Shoulder to Hand - Release Your Kinetic Chain by Dr. Brian Abelson and Kamali T. Abelson

If you suffer from Shoulder Pain, Golfers Elbow, Tennis Elbow, Rotator Cuff Syndrome, carpal tunnel syndrome, wrist pain, or other hand injuries, this book reveals how everything you do – from working at your desk, to swinging a golf club - impacts the complex kinetic chain relationships within your soft tissue structures. The exercises are designed to help build and strengthen these neuromuscular relationships – a key step to resolving long-standing soft-tissue injuries, and improving strength, power, and sports performance.

Available Now!

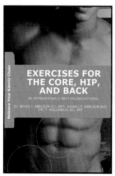

Kinetic Chain Exercises for Core, Hip, and Back - Release Your Kinetic Chain by Dr. Brian Abelson, Dr. Tarveen Ahluwalia, and Kamali T. Abelson

If you suffer from back pain, sciatica, or hip pain, have problems with core stability, or have the desire to improve your sports performance, then this is the book for you. Kinetic chain problems originating in the core are often the missing link for resolving chronic or acute injuries. This book takes you through a step-by-step process - from beginner to advanced - to release the power in your core and develop strength and flexibility without injury.

Coming Soon

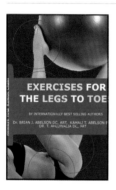

Kinetic Chain Exercise for the Hips to Toes - Release Your Kinetic Chain by Dr. Brian Abelson, Dr. Tarveen Ahluwalia, and Kamali T. Abelson

If you suffer from Plantar Fasciitis, Achilles Tendonitis, Iliotibial Band Syndrome, shin splints, knee pain, foot pain, or other lower extremity injuries then this book is for you. We considered key kinetic chain relationships in the development of each exercise routine in this book. Each routine helps strengthen key neuromuscular relationships – a key step in resolving long-standing soft-tissue injuries and in improving sports performance!

Coming Soon

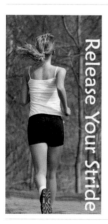

Release your Stride by Dr. Brian Abelson and Kamali T. Abelson

Runners, are you looking for a way to increase your running performance? Would you like to identify and correct those little biomechanical flaws that '*throw you off your stride*'?

This book gives you the tools you need to identify, correct, and resolve these problems, and get you performing at your best... whether you are a recreational runner or a professional athlete.

Coming Soon

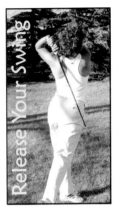

Notes

Notes

Notes

Notes